Uwe Frank   Evelina Tacconelli

The Daschner Guide to

In-Hospital Antibiotic Therapy

T0175248

**This useful "always on-hand" pocket guide
can easily be ordered:**
http://www.springer.com/978-3-642-18401-7

Uwe Frank   Evelina Tacconelli

The Daschner Guide to

In-Hospital Antibiotic Therapy

With 18 Figures and 6 Tables

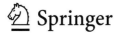

Uwe Frank, MD, PhD
Professor of Clinical Microbiology
Head, Division of Infection Control and Hospital Epidemiology
Department of Infectious Diseases
Heidelberg University Hospital
Im Neuenheimer Feld 324
69120 Heidelberg, Germany

Evelina Tacconelli, MD, PhD
Assistant Professor of Infectious Diseases
Institute of Infectious Diseases
Università Cattolica del Sacro Cuore
Largo Gemelli 8
00168 Rome, Italy

Library of Congress Control Number: 2011932844

ISBN 978-3-642-18401-7 Springer Medizin Verlag Heidelberg

Corrected printing 2012

Springer Medizin
Springer-Verlag GmbH
ein Unternehmen von Springer Science+Business
springer.com

© Springer Medizin Verlag Heidelberg 2012

Editor: Hinrich Küster
Project Mangement: Kerstin Barton
Cover Design: deblik Berlin, Germany
Typesetting: Fotosatz-Service Köhler GmbH, Würzburg, Germany

SPIN: 86058632

Printed on acid-free paper   2122 – 5 4 3 2 1

Foreword

Dear Colleagues,

Why another book on antibiotic therapy?

The answer might simply be that antibiotic therapy is a cornerstone of everybody's daily clinical experience.

Or that antimicrobial therapy is often a neglected area in both academic courses and continuous medical education.

Or that infections are the unwanted companion of so many and so diverse noninfectious diseases, and that an agile and multifaceted approach to antibiotic therapy cannot be but welcome by all those involved in the different medical and surgical disciplines.

Or that saving the antibiotic power through their judicious use must be supported at all costs in these difficult times.

Or possibly that all the aforementioned statements hold true, yet not exhausting the vast array of reasons that make this book timely, needed, and very welcome by so many.

A second and obvious question is whether the book by Frank and Tacconelli is up to the level and might aim at being a faithful companion for all those dealing with antimicrobial drugs. The answer can be found in the enduring success of its previous editions and in the enthusiasm with which the authors have updated and improved an already successful text.

The treatment of infections caused by Gram-positives is now discussed by including the most recent molecules, which are already playing a major role in many scenarios. Although there are fewer newly available for the treatment of infections caused by Gram-negatives, the available therapeutic choices are rediscussed and fine tuned in the light of the changing and worrisome epidemiology of bacterial resistance. Finally, antimycotics are extensively discussed so as to match the increasing challenge represented by fungal infections in most clinical settings.

All in all, this book looks towards a future in which antimicrobial resistance will certainly represent an ever-growing obstacle for medicine and for which books like this will undoubtedly represent a valuable resource.

Giuseppe Cornaglia, MD, PhD
President, European Society of Clinical Microbiology and Infectious Diseases (ESCMID)
Department of Pathology and Infection
University of Verona, Italy

Preface

The first edition of Franz Daschner's pocketbook "Antibiotika am Krankenbett" was published in Germany in 1982. The purpose of the book was to provide physicians and pharmacists, residents, medical students and healthcare professionals in allied fields with a concise reference source for antibiotic drugs, listing the preparations available, antimicrobial spectra, usual dosages, adverse effects, and, in specific cases pharmacologic data. The German book was regularly updated and its structure modified according to the users' needs. In 2009, we were asked to prepare a new version of the pocketbook in English, and because of the pocketbook's popularity among clinicians and pharmacists throughout Europe, we are proud to present today the completely revised and updated 2nd edition.

The book's pocket size has always been popular and we are committed to maintaining this design so that the book can be slipped into the pocket of any jacket or laboratory coat and carried throughout the hospital.

Changes in antibiotic therapy have evolved simultaneously with developing antibiotic resistance and new emerging pathogens. These developments are so rapid that no textbook of clinical microbiology, infectious diseases and pharmacology can keep pace. Clinicians nowadays rely on the medical literature to prescribe antibiotics, but concise information useful for patient management is often difficult to obtain. We believe that with respect to antibiotic therapy this handbook is unparalleled in its precision and conciseness. Its structure is designed for easy use. It attempts to present the most common trade names for antibiotics marketed in Europe and should be used only as a guideline to these. It should not be considered as an official therapeutic document. If there is any discrepancy between the recommendations made and the information available in the package inserts, the reader is advised to obtain official and complete information from the national office of the manufacturer.

If you wish to comment on or criticise any of the recommendations made in the pocketbook, please, e-mail us at the following addresses:

uwe.frank@med.uni-heidelberg.de
etacconelli@rm.unicatt.it

Please let us know if you notice that a particular antibiotic or pathogen has not been covered. Please also feel free to suggest experts who could contribute to the subject.
We look forward to hearing from you!

Uwe Frank   Evelina Tacconelli

Acknowledgements

Our thanks for helping to update the 2nd edition of "The Daschner Guide to In-Hospital Antibiotic Therapy" to:

Joachim Boehler, MD, PhD, Wiesbaden, Germany
Michela Cipriani, MD, Rome, Italy
Martin Hug, PhD, Freiburg, Germany
Manfred Kist, MD, PhD, Freiburg, Germany
Eva-Maria Kleissle, MD, Heidelberg, Germany
Lyubomira Rabadzhieva, MS, Freiburg, Germany

Contents

Abbreviations

Drug dosage and drug administration:

od	Once daily
bid	Two times daily
tid	Three times daily
qid	Four times daily
p.o.	Per os (by mouth)
i.v.	Intravenous
i.m.	Intramuscular

BAL	Bronchoalveolar lavage/tracheal wash
BW	Body weight
CAPD	Continuous ambulatory peritoneal dialysis
CAVH	Continuous arteriovenous haemofiltration
CNS	Central nervous system
Crea	Creatinine
CrCl	Creatinine clearance
CSF	Cerebrospinal fluid
CVC	Central venous catheter
CVVH/CVVHD	Continuous venovenous haemofiltration/ haemodialysis
DI	Dosage interval
div	Divided
ESBL	Extended-spectrum beta-lactamases
GFR	Glomerular filtration rate
GISA	Glycopeptide intermediate-resistant *S. aureus*
HD	Haemodialysis
INH	Isoniazid
IU	International unit
LD	Loading dose
MAO	Monoamine oxidase
MDR	Multidrug resistant
MRSA	Methicillin-resistant *S. aureus*

MRSE	Methicillin-resistant *S. epidermidis*
MSSA	Methicillin-sensitive *S. aureus*
NB	Nota bene
TMP/SMX	Trimethoprim-sulfamethoxazole
UTI	Urinary tract infection
VRE	Vancomycin-resistant enterococci

The Authors

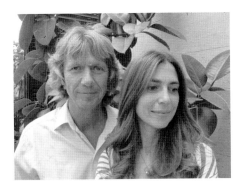

Uwe Frank, MD, PhD, is a Professor of Clinical Microbiology at the University of Heidelberg, Department of Infectious Diseases, Heidelberg University Hospital and a Senior Lecturer on Infection Control and Hospital Epidemiology at the University of Freiburg, Department of Environmental Health Sciences, Freiburg University Hospital, Germany. He was a work package leader in the European IPSE/HELICS project (Improving Patient Safety in Europe/Hospital in Europe Link for Infection Control through Surveillance), coordinator of the BURDEN project (Burden of Resistance and Disease in European Nations), and is currently coordinator of the IMPLEMENT project (Implementing Strategic Bundles for Infection Prevention and Management), which were all financed by the EU Commission Directorate-General for Health and Consumer Protection (DG SANCO).

Evelina Tacconelli, MD, PhD, is an Assistant Professor of Infectious Diseases at the Università Cattolica Sacro Cuore, Rome, Italy. She has been a Lecturer on Medicine at the Beth Israel Deaconess Medical Center and Harvard Medical School, Boston, USA. She was the recipient of awards from the European Society of Clinical Microbiology and Infectious Diseases

(ESCMID) for research excellence. She is the ESCMID Professional Affair Officer for Infectious Diseases and serves on the editorial board of Clinical Microbiology and Infection. She is a work package leader in the European SATURN project (Impact of Specific Antibiotic Therapies on the Prevalence of Human Host Resistant Bacteria, 7th framework) and in the IMPLEMENT project (DG SANCO).

1 Classification of the Antibiotics

β-Lactam antibiotics

Benzylpenicillins	Phenoxy-penicillins (oral penicillins)	Penicillinase-resistant penicillins (anti-staphylococcal penicillins)
Penicillin G (benzylpenicillin sodium, procaine benzylpenicillin, benzathine penicillin)	Penicillin V Propicillin	Oxacillin Dicloxacillin Flucloxacillin
Aminobenzyl-penicillins	**Ureidopenicillins (broad-spectrum penicillins)**	**ß-Lactam/ ß-lactamase inhibitors**
Ampicillin Amoxicillin	Mezlocillin Piperacillin	Ampicillin/ sulbactam Amoxicillin/ clavulanate Piperacillin/ tazobactam Sulbactam in free combinations

Cephalosporins (first generation)	Cephalosporins (second generation)	Cephalosporins (third and fourth generation)
Cefazolin	Cefuroxime	Cefotaxime
Cefalexin (oral)	Cefotiam	Ceftriaxone
Cefadroxil (oral)	Cefuroxime axetil	Ceftazidime
	Cefaclor (oral)	Cefepime
	Loracarbef	Cefixime (oral)
		Cefpodoxime proxetil (oral)
		Ceftibuten (oral)

Monobactams	Carbapenems	β-Lactamase inhibitors
Aztreonam	Imipenem	Clavulanic acid
	Meropenem	Sulbactam
	Ertapenem	Tazobactam
	Doripenem	

Other substances

Aminoglycosides	Tetracyclines	Quinolones
Streptomycin	Tetracycline	Group I:
Gentamicin	Doxycycline	Norfloxacin
Tobramycin	Minocycline	
Netilmicin		Group II:
Amikacin		Enoxacin
		Ofloxacin
		Ciprofloxacin
		Group III:
		Levofloxacin
		Group IV:
		Moxifloxacin

I: Indications essentially limited to UTI

II: Widely indicated

III: Improved activity against Gram-positive and atypical
      pathogens

IV: Further enhanced activity against Gram-positive and
      atypical pathogens, also against anaerobic bacteria

Lincosamides	**Azol derivatives**	**Nitroimidazoles**
Clindamycin	Miconazole	Metronidazole
	Ketoconazole	
	Fluconazole	
	Itraconazole	
	Voriconazole	
	Posaconazole	

Glycopeptide antibiotics	**Macrolides**	**Polyenes**
Vancomycin	Erythromycin	Amphotericin B
Teicoplanin	Spiramycin	Nystatin
Telavancin	Roxithromycin	
	Clarithromycin	
	Azithromycin	

Glycylcyclines		**Echinocandins**
Tigecycline		Caspofungin
		Anidulafungin
		Micafungin

Streptogramines	**Ketolides**	**Oxazolidinones**
Quinupristin/ dalfopristin	Telithromycin	Linezolid

Lipopeptides

Daptomycin

Epoxides

Fosfomycin

Polymyxins

Colistin
(polymyxin E)
Polymyxin B

Ansamycins

Rifampicin

2 Antibiotics Marketed in the EU

Generics and Trade Names

Generics	Trade Names (Selection)	Page
Amikacin	Amicasil® (GR, IT), Amikacin® (DE), Amikaver® (TR), Amikin® (CZ, GB, HR, HU, PL), Amiklin® (FR), Amukin® (BE, NL), BB K8® (IT), Biclin® (ES, PT), Biklin® (AT, DK, FI, SE)	77
Amoxicillin	Amox® (IT), Actimoxi® (ES), Agram® (FR), Aktil® (HU), Alfoxil® (TR), Almacin® (HR), Almodan® (GB), Amimox® (NO, SE), Amoclen® (CZ), Amorion® (FI), Amotaks® (PL), Amoxi® (BE), Amoxillin® (NO), Amoxypen® (DE)	79
Amoxicillin/ clavulanate	Abba® (IT), Aktil® (HU), Amiclav® (GB), Amoclan® (AT, NL), Amoclavam® (PT), Amoklavin® (TR), Amoxi comp® (FI), Augmentan® (DE), Augmentin® (BE, CZ, PL), Clamoxyl® (ES)	80
Amphotericin B	Amphocycline® (FR), Ampho-Moronal® (AT, DE), Amphotericin B® (DE), Fungilin® (DK, GB), Fungizona® (ES), Fungizone® (FI, IT, NO, NL, SE)	81
Amphotericin B (liposomal)	AmBisome (DE, ES, FR, GB, IT)	82

Generics	Trade Names (Selection)	Page
Ampicillin	Abetathen® (GR), Alongamicina® (ES), Amfipen® (GB), Amplital® (IT), Ampicillin® (DE, HU), Ampicin® (FI), Amplifar® (PT), Binotal® (AT), Doktacilin® (DK, NO, S), Fortapen® (BE), Penbritin® (BE, HR, NL), Totapen® (FR)	83
Ampicillin/ sulbactam (Sultamicillin)	Alfasid® (TR), Begalin® (GR), Unacid® (DE, PT), Unacim® (FR), Unasyn® (AT, CZ, DE, ES, GB, IT, PL)	84
Anidulafungin	Ecalta® (AT, DE, DK, ES, FI, FR, GB, IS, NO, SE)	86
Azithromycin	Azitromax® (NO, S), Azitrox® (CZ, PL), Zithromax® (AT, BE, DE, ES, FI, FR, GB, GR, NL, PT), Zitromax® (DK, IT, TR)	87
Aztreonam	Azactam® (AT, BE, CZ, DE, DK, ES, FI, FR, GB, GR, IT, NL, NO, PT, PL, S, TR), Primbactam® (IT)	88
Caspofungin	Cancidas® (AT, BE, CZ, DE, DK, ES, FI, FR, GB, IT, NL, NO, PL, S)	89
Cefaclor	Alfatil® (FR), Altaclor® (IT), Bacticlor® (GB), Ceclor® (AT, BE, CZ, ES, GR, HR, HU, NL, PL, PT, TR), Panoral® (DE)	90
Cefadroxil	Baxan® (GB), Biodroxil® (AT, CZ, GR, PL, PT), Cefadril® (IT), Cefamox® (S), Cefroxil® (ES), Duracef® (BE, FI, HR, HU), Grüncef® (DE), Moxacef® (BE, GR, NL), Oracéfal® (FR)	91

Generics	Trade Names (Selection)	Page
Cefalexin	Cefalexina® (IT), Cefaclen® (CZ), Cefadina® (ES), Cefalin® (FR, HR), Cephalexin® (DE), Ceporex® (BE, FR), Kefalex® (FI), Keflex® (AT, DK, GB, GR, NO, PL, PT, S), Keforal® (NL)	92
Cefazolin	Areuzolin® (ES), Biofazolin® (PL), Biozolin® (GR) Céfacidal® (BE, FR, NL), Cefamezin® (PT, TR), Cefazil® (IT), Cephazolin fresenius® (DE), Kefzol® (AT, BE, CZ, HR, NL, TR)	93
Cefepime	Axepim® (FR), Maxipime® (AT, BE, CZ, DE, ES, FI, GR, HR, IT, NL, PL, PT, S, TR)	94
Cefixime	Aerocef® (AT), Bonocef® (PT), Ceftoral® (GR), Cephoral® (DE), Denvar® (ES), Oroken® (FR), Supracef® (FI), Suprax® (CZ, HU, IT, GB, TR), Tricef® (SE)	96
Cefotaxime	Biotaksym® (PL), Claforan® (AT, BE, CZ, DE, DK, ES, IT, FI, FR, GB, GR, HU, NL, NO, SE, TR)	97
Cefotiam	Halospor® (AT), Spizef® (AT, DE), Taketiam® (FR)	98
Cefpodoxime proxetil	Biocef® (AT), Orelox® (CZ, DE, DK, ES, FR, GB, GR, IT, NL, SE)	99
Ceftazidime	Cefortam® (PT), Ceftazidim® (DE), Fortam® (ES), Fortum® (AT, CZ, DE, DK, FR, GB, NL, NO, PL, SE, TR), Ftazidime® (GR), Glazidim® (BE, FI, IT)	100

Generics	Trade Names (Selection)	Page
Ceftibuten	Biocef® (ES), Caedax® (AT, GR, PT), Cedax® (ES, HR, HU, IT, NL, PL, SE), Keimax® (DE)	101
Ceftriaxone	Axobat® (IT), Lendacin® (CZ) Rocefalin® (ES), Rocefin® (IT), Rocephalin® (DK, FI, NO, SE), Rocephin® (AT, DE, GB, GR, HR, NL, PL, PT, TR), Rocéphine® (BE, FR)	102
Cefuroxime	Cecim® (HU), Cefurin® (IT), Curoxima® (ES), Ketocef® (HR), Zinacef® (BE, CZ, DE, DK, FI, GB, GR, NL, NO, PL, SE, TR)	104
Cefuroxime axetil	Cefurobac® (AT), Cepazine® (FR), Elobact® (DE), Interbion® (GR) Zinnat® (AT, BE, CZ, DK, ES, FI, FR, GB, HR, HU, IT, NL, PL, SE, TR)	105
Chloramphenicol	Chlorocid® (HU), Chloromycetin® (AT, DK, ES, FI, GB, PT, SE), Cloramfenicolo® (IT), Cloranic® (GR), Globenicol® (NL)	106
Ciprofloxacin	Aceoto® (ES), Carmicina® (PT), Ciproxin® (IT), Cilox® (NO), Ciprinol® (CZ, HR, PL), Ciprobay® (CZ, DE, HU, PL)	107
Clarithromycin	Biclar® (BE), Claromycin® (GR), Klacid® (AT, CZ, DE, DK, ES, FI, HR, IT, NL, NO, PL, PT, SE, TR)	109
Clindamycin	Cleocin® (TR), Dalacin® C (AT, BE, CZ, DK, FI, GB, HU, IT, NL, NO, PL, SE), Sobelin® (DE)	110

Generics	Trade Names (Selection)	Page
Colistin	Colimicina® (IT, ES), Colimycin® (DK, NO), Colimycine® (BE, FR), Colistin® (AT, DE, GR, PL), Colomycin® (GB)	111
Cotrimoxazole	Abactrim® (ES), Bactrim® (AT, BE, CZ, DK, FI, FR, GB, IT, NO, PL, PT, SE, TR), Eusaprim® (AT, BE, DE, IT, NL, SE)	112
Daptomycin	Cubicin® (AT, DE, ES, FR, GB, IT, NO, PT, SE)	114
Dicloxacillin	Diclocil® (DK, FI, GR, NL, NO, PT, SE)	115
Doripenem	Doribax® (AT, DE, ES, FI, GB, NO, SE)	116
Doxycycline	Actidox® (PT), Bassado® (IT), Clisemina® (ES), Dinamisin® (TR), Dotur® (PL), Doxy® (BE, FR), Doxy-hexal® (DE), Vibramycin® (AT, CZ, DK, GB, GR, HR, NO, NL, SE)	117
Enoxacin	Comprecin® (GB), Enoksetin® (TR), Enoxabion® (FI), Enoxen® (IT), Enoxor® (AT, DE, FR), Gyramid® (CZ)	118
Ertapenem	Invanz® (AT, CZ, DE, DK, ES, FR, FI, GB, HR, IT, NO, PL, SE)	119
Erythromycin	Abboticin® (DK, FI, NO, SE), Bronse-ma® (ES), Eritrocina (IT), Erythrocin® (AT, CZ, DE, GB, GR, TR), Érythrocine® (BE, FR, NL)	120

Generics	Trade Names (Selection)	Page
Ethambutol	Clobutol® (PT), EMB-Fatol® (AT, DE), Embutol® (TR), Etapiam® (IT), Myambutol® (AT, BE, DE, DK, ES, GB, GR, FR, NL), Oributol® (FI), Sural® (CZ, HU)	121
Flucloxacillin	Flix® (TR), Floxapen® (AT, BE, GB, GR, NL, NO, PT), Flucinal® (IT), Heracillin® (DK, SE), Pantaflux® (IT), Staphylex® (DE, FI)	122
Fluconazole	Diflucan® (AT, BE, CZ, DE, DK, ES, IT, FI, GB, HR, HU, NL, NO, PL, PT, SE), Tierlite® (GR), Triflucan® (FR, TR)	123
Flucytosine	Ancotil® (AT, CZ, DE, DK, ES, FI, FR, GB, IT, NL, NO, PL, PT, SE)	125
Fosfomycin	Fosfocin® (DK, IT), Infectofos® (DE)	127
Gentamicin	Cidomycin® (GB), Garamycin® (CZ, DK, FI, GR, HR, NL, NO, PL, SE, TR), Gentamicina® (IT), Refobacin® (DE)	129
Imipenem/cilastatin	Primaxin® (GB, GR), Tienam® (BE, CZ, DK, ES, FI, FR, HR, IT, NL, NO, PL, PT, SE, TR), Zienam® (DE, AT)	130
Isoniazid (INH)	Eutizon® (HR), Isoniazid® (HU), Isozid® (DE), Nicozid® (IT), Nidrazid® (CZ), Rimifon® (BE, FR, GB)	132
Itraconazole	Canadiol® (ES), Funit® (TR), Itrac® (HR), Orungal® (HU, PL), Sempera® (DE), Sporanox® (AT, BE, CZ, DK, FI, FR, GB, GR, IT, NO, PT, SE)	133

Generics	Trade Names (Selection)	Page
Levofloxacin	Tavanic® (AT, BE, CZ, DE, ES, FI, FR, GB, GR, HR, IT, NL, PL, PT, SE, TR)	134
Linezolid	Zyvox® (GB), Zyvoxid® (AT, BE, CZ, DE, DK, ES, FI, FR, IT, NL, NO, PL, PT, SE)	135
Loracarbef	Lorabid® (AT, GR, NL, SE, TR), Lorafem® (DE)	136
Meropenem	Merinfec® (AT), Meronem® (BE, CZ, DE, DK, ES, FI, GB, GR, HR, HU, NL, NO, PL, PT, SE, TR), Merrem® (IT)	137
Metronidazole	Alvidral® (GR), Amotein® (ES), Anaeromet® (BE), Clont® (DE), Defla-mon® (IT), Dumozol® (PT), Efloran® (CZ, HR), Elyzol® (AT, DK, FI, FR, GB, NL, NO, SE)	138
Mezlocillin	Baypen® (AT, DE, FR, GB, IT, SE, TR)	139
Micafungin	Mycamine® (DE, IT)	140
Minocycline	Logryx® (FR), Minocin® (AT, BE, ES, GB, GR, IT, PT), Minocyclin® (DE)	141
Moxifloxacin	Actira® (AT, DE, ES), Avalox® (AT, BE, CZ, DE, DK, FI, GB, GR, HR, IT, NL, PL, PT, SE, TR), Izilox® (FR)	142
Netilmicin	Certomycin® (AT), Netilin® (GB), Netrocin® (ES), Netromicina® (PT), Netromicine® (BE, CZ, FR, HR, NL, PL, TR), Netromycin® (GR), Nettacin® (IT), Netylin® (DK, FI, NO, SE)	143

Generics	Trade Names (Selection)	Page
Nitrofurantoin	Furadantin® (AT, GB, IT, NO, SE), Furadantina® (PT), Furadantine® (BE, FR, NL), Furantonin® (CZ), Furantoina® (ES), Furedan® (IT), Furolin® (GR), Macrofuran® (FI), Nifurantin® (DE), Ninur® (HR), Piyeloseptyl® (TR), Siraliden® (PL)	145
Norfloxacin	Alenbit® (GR), Amicrobin® (ES), Barazan® (DE), Chibroxol® (BE, NL, PT), Diperflox® (IT), Floxacin® (AT), Gyrablock® (CZ), Lexinor® (FI, SE), Noroxin® (ES, FR, GB, IT, NL, PT, TR), Zoroxin® (AT, BE, DK)	145
Nystatin	Fungicidin® (CZ), Fungostatin® (TR), Macmiror® (CZ, PL, TR), Moronal® (DE), Mycostatin® (AT, BE, DK, ES, FI, FR, GR, IT, NO, PT, SE), Nystan® (GB)	146
Ofloxacin	Docofloxacine® (BE), Oflocin® (IT), Tarivid® (DE)	147
Oxacillin	Bristopen® (FR), InfectoStaph® (DE), Oxacillin® (CZ), Penstapho® (BE, IT), Stapenor® (AT)	147
Penicillin G (Benzyl-penicillin)	Omnacilina® (PT), Penicillin Gruenenthal® (DE), Penidural® (GB, NL), Peniroger® (ES)	149
Penicillin V (Phenoxy-methylpenicillin)	Isocillin (DE), Megacillin oral (DE) and other in DE, Oracilline (FR), Phenoxymethylpenicillin (GB)	151
Pentamidine isethionate	Pentacarinat® (DE, ES, GR, FR, GB, GR, IT, NO)	215

Generics	Trade Names (Selection)	Page
Piperacillin	Avocin® (IT), Piperacillin® (DE), Piperilline® (FR), Piperital® (IT) Pipraks® (TR), Pipril® (AT, CZ, ES, FI, GB, GR, HR, PT)	152
Piperacillin/ Tazobactam	Tazobac® (DE), Tazocel® (ES), Tazocilline® (FR), Tazocin® (BE, DK, GB, HU, IT, NL, NO, PL, SE, TR)	153
Posaconazole	Noxafil® (AT, DE, DK, ES, FR, GB, IT, NO, SE)	154
Protionamide	Ektebin® (DE), Isoprodian® (AT), Promid® (TR), Tebeform® (HU), Trevintix® (GB)	155
Pyrazinamide	Piraldina® (IT, TR), Pyrafat® (DE, AT), Tebrazid® (BE), Tisamid® (CZ, FI)	156
Quinupristin/ dalfopristin	Synercid® (AT, CZ, DE, ES, FR, GB, IT, PL)	157
Rifabutin	Ansatipine® (ES, FI, FR, SE), Mycobutin® (AT, BE, CZ, DE, GB, GR, IT, NL, PT, TR)	158
Rifampin/ Rifampicin	Arficin® (CZ, HR), Eremfat® (AT, DE), Rifadin® (GB, GR, IT, NL, PT, SE, TR), Rifarm® (FI), Rimactan® (BE, DK, ES, FR, NO, SE), Tubocin® (HU)	159
Rifampin + Isoniazid	Rifinah® (DE, FR, GB, GR, IT, NL, PT, TR), Rifamazid® (PL), Rimactazid® (DK, NO, SE)	160
Rifampin + Isoniazid + Pyrazinamide	Rifater® (AT, DE, ES, FR, GB, IT, PT, TR), Rimcure® (NO, SE)	160

Generics	Trade Names (Selection)	Page
Rifampin + Isoniazid + Pyrazinamide + Ethambutol	Rimstar (DK, NO, SE)	160
Roxithromycin	Acevor® (GB, GR), Roxithromycin® (DE), Rulid® (BE, CZ, FR, GR, IT, PL, TR), Rulide® (AT, ES, NL, PT), Surlid® (DK, FI, SE)	160
Spiramycin	Rovamicina (IT), Rovamycine (AT, BE, CZ, DE, FR, GR, HR, HU, NL, PL, TR)	224
Streptomycin	Estreptomicina® (ES), Pan-Streptomycin® (GR), Strep-Deva® (TR), Streptomicina® (IT), Streptomycin® (DE)	161
Sulbactam	Betamaze® (FR), Combactam® (DE, AT)	162
Sultamicillin	(see Ampicillin/Sulbactam)	84
Teicoplanin	Targocid® (AT, BE, CZ, DE, DK, ES, FI, FR, GB, GR, HR, NL, NO, PL, SE, TR), Targosid® (IT, PT)	164
Telavancin	Vibativ® (Marketing application submitted)	268
Telithromycin	Ketek® (AT, BE, DE, ES, FI, FR, GB, HR, IT, NO, PL, PT, SE)	165
Tetracycline	Chropicyclin® (GR), Ciclobiotico® (PT), Tetracyclin® (DE), Tetralysal® (AT, BE, CZ, DK, ES, FI, FR, GB, IT, NO, PL, SE), Tetrarco® (NL)	166

Generics	Trade Names (Selection)	Page
Tigecycline	Tygacil® (AT, CZ, DE, ES, FR, GB, IT, NO, SE)	167
Tobramycin	Bramicil® (IT), Bramitob® (GB, NL), Brulamycin® (AT, CZ, HU), Distobram® (PT), Gernebcin® (DE), Nebcin® (HR, TR), Nebcina® (DK, FI, NO, SE), Nebcine® (FR), Obracin® (BE), TOBI® (DE, FR, GB, PL)	168
Vancomycin	Diatracin® (ES), Edicin® (CZ, HR, HU, PL), Orivan® (FI), Vancocin® (AT, BE, GB, NL, PL, SE, TR), Vancocina® (IT)	169
Voriconazole	Vfend® (AT, BE, DE, CZ, DK, ES, FI, GB, IT, NL, NO, PL, PT, SE)	171

Trade Names and Generics

Trade Names (Selection)	Generics	Page
Abactrim® (ES)	Cotrimoxazole	112
Abba® (IT)	Amoxicillin/Clavulanate	80
Abboticin® (DK, FI, NO, SE)	Erythromycin	120
Abetathen® (GR)	Ampicillin	83
Aceoto® (ES)	Ciprofloxacin	107
Acevor® (GB, GR)	Roxithromycin	158
Actidox® (PT)	Doxycycline	117
Actimoxi® (ES)	Amoxicillin	79
Actira® (AT, ES, DE)	Moxifloxacin	142

Trade Names (Selection)	Generics	Page
Aerocef® (AT)	Cefixime	96
Agram® (FR)	Amoxicillin	79
Aktil® (HU)	Amoxicillin	79
Alenbit® (GR)	Norfloxacin	145
Alfasid® (TR)	Ampicillin/Sulbactam	84
Alfatil® (FR)	Cefaclor	90
Alfoxil® (TR)	Amoxicillin	79
Almacin® (HR)	Amoxicillin	79
Almodan® (GB)	Amoxicillin	79
Alongamicina® (ES)	Ampicillin	83
Altaclor® (IT)	Cefaclor	90
Alvidral® (GR)	Metronidazole	138
Amfipen® (GB)	Ampicillin	83
Amicasil® (GR, IT)	Amikacin	77
Amiclav® (GB)	Amoxicillin/Clavulanate	80
Amicrobin® (ES)	Norfloxacin	145
Amikacin® (DE)	Amikacin	77
Amikaver® (TR)	Amikacin	77
Amikin® (CZ, GB, HR, HU, PL)	Amikacin	77
Amiklin® (FR)	Amikacin	77
Amimox® (NO, SE)	Amoxicillin	79

Trade Names (Selection)	Generics	Page
Amoclan® (AT, NL)	Amoxicillin/Clavulanate	80
Amoclavam® (PT)	Amoxicillin/Clavulanate	80
Amoclen® (CZ)	Amoxicillin	79
Amoklavin® (TR)	Amoxicillin/Clavulanate	80
Amorion® (FI)	Amoxicillin	79
Amotaks® (PL)	Amoxicillin	79
Amotein® (ES)	Metronidazole	138
Amox® (IT)	Amoxicillin	79
Amoxi® (BE)	Amoxicillin	79
Amoxi comp® (FI)	Amoxicillin/Clavulanate	80
Amoxillin® (NO)	Amoxicillin	79
Amoxypen® (DE)	Amoxicillin	79
Amphocycline® (FR)	Amphotericin B	81
Ampicin® (FI)	Ampicillin	84
Ampho-Moronal® (AT, DE)	Amphotericin B	81
Amphotericin B® (DE)	Amphotericin B	81
Ampicillin® (DE, HU)	Ampicillin	83
Amplifar® (PT)	Ampicillin	83
Amplital® (IT)	Ampicillin	83
Amukin® (BE, NL)	Amikacin	77

Trade Names (Selection)	Generics	Page
Anaeromet® (BE)	Metronidazole	138
Ancotil® (AT, CZ, DE, DK, ES, FI, FR, GB, IT, NL, NO, PL, PT, SE)	Flucytosine	125
Ansatipine® (ES, FI, FR, SE)	Rifabutin	158
Areuzolin® (ES)	Cefazolin	93
Arficin® (CZ, HR)	Rifampicin	159
Augmentan® (DE),	Amoxicillin/Clavulanate	80
Augmentin® (BE, CZ, PL)	Amoxicillin/Clavulanate	80
Avalox® (AT, BE, CZ, DE, DK, FI, GB, GR, HR, IT, NL, PL, PT, SE, TR)	Moxifloxacin	142
Avocin® (IT)	Piperacillin	152
Axepim® (FR)	Cefepime	94
Axobat® (IT)	Ceftriaxone	102
Azactam® (AT, BE, CZ, DE, DK, ES, FR, FI, GB, GR, IT, NO, NL, PT, PL, SE, TR)	Aztreonam	88
Azitromax® (NO, SE)	Azithromycin	87
Azitrox® (CZ, PL)	Azithromycin	87
Bacticlor® (GB)	Cefaclor	90

Trade Names (Selection)	Generics	Page
Bactrim® (AT, BE, CZ, DK, FR, FI, GB, IT, NO, PT, PL, SE, TR)	Cotrimoxazole	112
Barazan® (DE)	Norfloxacin	145
Bassado® (IT)	Doxycycline	117
Baxan® (GB)	Cefadroxil	91
Baypen® (AT, DE, FR, GB, IT, SE, TR)	Mezlocillin	139
BB K8® (IT)	Amikacin	77
Begalin® (GR)	Ampicillin/Sulbactam	84
Betamaze® (FR)	Sulbactam	162
Biclar® (BE)	Clarithromycin	109
Biclin® (ES, PT)	Amikacin	77
Biklin® (AT, DK, FI, SE)	Amikacin	77
Biocef® (AT, ES)	Cefpodoxime proxetil Ceftibuten	99 101
Biotaksym® (PL)	Cefotaxime	97
Bonocef® (PT)	Cefixime	96
Binotal® (AT)	Ampicillin	83
Biodroxil® (AT, CZ, GR, PL, PT)	Cefadroxil	91
Biofazolin® (PL)	Cefazolin	93
Biozolin® (GR)	Cefazolin	93

Trade Names (Selection)	Generics	Page
Bramicil® (IT)	Tobramycin	168
Bramitob® (GB, NL)	Tobramycin	168
Bristopen® (FR)	Oxacillin	148
Bronsema® (ES)	Erythromycin	120
Brulamycin® (AT, CZ, HU)	Tobramycin	168
Canadiol® (ES)	Itraconazole	133
Cancidas® (AT, BE, CZ, DE, DK,ES, FI, FR, GB, IT, NO, NL, PL, SE)	Caspofungin	89
Carmicina® (PT)	Ciprofloxacin	107
Cecim® (HU)	Cefuroxime	104
Ceclor® (AT, BE, CZ, ES, GR, HR, HU, NL, PL, PT, TR)	Cefaclor	90
Caedax® (AT, GR, PT)	Ceftibuten	101
Cedax® (ES, HR, HU, IT, NL, PL, SE)	Ceftibuten	101
Cefaclen® (CZ)	Cefalexin	92
Céfacidal® (BE, FR, NL)	Cefazolin	93
Cefadina® (ES)	Cefalexin	92
Cefadril® (IT)	Cefadroxil	91
Cefalin® (FR, HR)	Cefalexin	92
Cefalexina (IT)	Cefalexin	92

Trade Names (Selection)	Generics	Page
Cefamezin® (PT, TR)	Cefazolin	93
Cefamox® (SE)	Cefadroxil	91
Cefazil (IT)	Cefazolin	93
Cefortam® (PT)	Ceftazidime	100
Cefroxil® (ES)	Cefadroxil	91
Ceftazidim® (DE)	Ceftazidime	100
Ceftoral® (GR)	Cefixime	96
Cefurin® (IT)	Cefuroxime	104
Cefurobac® (AT)	Cefuroxime-axetil	105
Cepazine® (FR)	Cefuroxime-axetil	105
Cephalexin® (DE)	Cefalexin	92
Cephazolin fresenius® (DE)	Cefazolin	93
Cephoral® (DE)	Cefixime	96
Ceporex® (BE, FR)	Cefalexin	92
Certomycin® (AT)	Netilmicin	143
Chibroxol® (BE, NL, PT)	Norfloxacin	145
Chlorocid® (HU)	Chloramphenicol	106
Chloromycetin® (AT, DK, ES, FI, GB, IT, PT, SE)	Chloramphenicol	106
Chropicyclin® (GR)	Tetracycline	166
Ciclobiotico® (PT)	Tetracycline	166

Trade Names (Selection)	Generics	Page
Cidomycin® (GB)	Gentamicin	129
Cilox® (NO)	Ciprofloxacin	107
Ciprinol® (CZ, HR, PL)	Ciprofloxacin	107
Ciprobay® (CZ, DE, HU, PL)	Ciprofloxacin	107
Ciproxin® (IT)	Ciprofloxacin	107
Claforan® (AT, BE, CZ, DE, DK, ES, GB, IT, FI, FR, GR, HU, NL, NO, SE, TR)	Cefotaxime	97
Clamoxyl® (ES)	Amoxicillin/Clavulanate	80
Claromycin® (GR)	Clarithromycin	109
Cleocin® (TR)	Clindamycin	110
Clobutol® (PT)	Ethambutol	121
Clont® (DE)	Metronidazole	138
Cloramfenicolo® (IT)	Chloramphenicol	106
Cloranic® (GR)	Chloramphenicol	106
Clisemina® (ES)	Doxycycline	117
Colimicina® (ES, IT)	Colistin	111
Colimycin® (DK, NO)	Colistin	111
Colimycine® (BE, FR)	Colistin	111
Colistin® (AT, DE, GR, PL)	Colistin	111
Colomycin® (GB)	Colistin	111
Combactam® (AT, DE)	Sulbactam	162

Trade Names (Selection)	Generics	Page
Comprecin® (GB)	Enoxacin	118
Cubicin® (AT, DE, ES, FR, GB, IT, NO, PT, SE)	Daptomycin	114
Curoxima® (ES)	Cefuroxime	104
Dalacin® C (AT, BE, CZ, DK, FI, GB, HU, IT, NL, NO, PL, SE)	Clindamycin	110
Deflamon® (IT)	Metronidazole	138
Denvar® (ES)	Cefixime	96
Diatracin® (ES)	Vancomycin	169
Dicapen® (GB)	Ampicillin/Sulbactam	84
Diclocil® (DK, FI, GR, NL, NO, PT, SE)	Dicloxacillin	115
Diflucan® (AT, BE, CZ, DE, DK, ES, GB, IT, FI, HR, HU, NL, NO, PL, PT, SE)	Fluconazole	123
Dinamisin® (TR)	Doxycycline	117
Diperflox® (IT)	Norfloxacin	145
Distobram® (PT)	Tobramycin	168
Docofloxacine® (BE)	Ofloxacin	147
Doktacilin® (DK, NO, SE)	Ampicillin	83
Doribax® (AT, DE, ES, FI, GB, NO, SE)	Doripenem	116
Dotur® (PL)	Doxycycline	117

Trade Names (Selection)	Generics	Page
Doxy® (BE, FR)	Doxycycline	117
Doxyhexal® (DE)	Doxycycline	117
Dumozol® (PT)	Metronidazole	138
Duracef® (BE, FI, HR, HU)	Cefadroxil	91
Ecalta® (AT, DE, DK, ES, FI, FR, GB, IS, NO, SE)	Anidulafungin	86
Edicin® (CZ, HR, HU, PL)	Vancomycin	169
Efloran® (CZ, HR)	Metronidazole	138
Ektebin® (DE)	Protionamide	155
Elobact® (DE)	Cefuroxime axetil	105
Elyzol® (AT, DK, FI, FR, GB, NL, NO, SE)	Metronidazole	138
EMB-Fatol® (AT, DE)	Ethambutol	121
Embutol® (TR)	Ethambutol	121
Enoksetin® (TR)	Enoxacin	118
Enoxabion® (FI)	Enoxacin	118
Enoxen® (IT)	Enoxacin	118
Enoxor® (AT, DE, FR)	Enoxacin	118
Eremfat® (AT, DE)	Rifampicin	159
Eritrocina® (IT)	Erythromycin	120
Erythrocin® (AT, CZ, DE, GB, GR, TR)	Erythromycin	120
Érythrocine® (BE, FR, NL)	Erythromycin	120

Trade Names (Selection)	Generics	Page
Estreptomicina® (ES)	Streptomycin	161
Etapiam® (IT)	Ethambutol	121
Eusaprim® (AT, BE, DE, IT, NL, SE)	Cotrimoxazole	112
Eutizon® (HR)	Isoniazid (INH)	132
Flix® (TR)	Flucloxacillin	122
Floxacin® (AT)	Norfloxacin	145
Floxapen® (AT, BE, GB, GR, NL, NO,PT)	Flucloxacillin	122
Flucinal® (IT)	Flucloxacillin	122
Fortam® (ES)	Ceftazidime	100
Fortapen® (BE)	Ampicillin	83
Fortum® (AT, CZ, DE, DK, FR, GB, NL, NO, PL, SE, TR)	Ceftazidime	100
Fosfocin® (DK, IT)	Fosfomycin	127
Ftazidime® (GR)	Ceftazidime	100
Fungicidin® (CZ)	Nystatin	146
Fungilin® (DK, GB)	Amphotericin B	81
Fungizona® (ES)	Amphotericin B	81
Fungizone® (FI, IT, NL, NO, SE)	Amphotericin B	81
Fungostatin® (TR)	Nystatin	146

Trade Names (Selection)	Generics	Page
Funit® (TR)	Itraconazole	133
Furadantin® (AT, GB, IT, NO, SE)	Nitrofurantoin	145
Furadantina® (PT)	Nitrofurantoin	145
Furadantine® (BE, FR, NL)	Nitrofurantoin	145
Furantoin® (CZ)	Nitrofurantoin	145
Furantoina® (ES)	Nitrofurantoin	145
Furedan® (IT)	Nitrofurantoin	145
Furolin® (GR)	Nitrofurantoin	145
Garamycin® (CZ, DK, FI, GR, HR, NL, NO, PL, SE, TR)	Gentamicin	129
Gentamicina® (IT)	Gentamicin	129
Gernebcin® (DE)	Tobramycin	168
Glazidim® (BE, FI, IT)	Ceftazidime	100
Globenicol® (NL)	Chloramphenicol	106
Grüncef® (DE)	Cefadroxil	91
Gyrablock® (CZ)	Norfloxacin	145
Gyramid® (CZ)	Enoxacin	118
Halospor® (AT)	Cefotiam	98
Heracillin® (DK, SE)	Flucloxacillin	122
Infectofos® (DE)	Fosfomycin	127
InfectoStaph® (DE)	Oxacillin	148

Trade Names (Selection)	Generics	Page
Interbion® (GR)	Cefuroxime axetil	105
Invanz® (AT, CZ, DE, DK, ES, FI, FR, GB, HR, IT, NO, PL, SE)	Ertapenem	119
Isocillin® (DE)	Penicillin V	151
Isoniazid® (HU)	Isoniazid (INH)	132
Isoprodian® (AT)	Protionamide	155
Isozid® (DE)	Isoniazid (INH)	132
Itrac® (HR)	Itraconazole	133
Izilox® (FR)	Moxifloxacin	142
Kefalex® (FI)	Cefadroxil	92
Keflex® (AT, DK, GB, GR, NO, PL, PT, SE)	Cefalexin	92
Keforal® (NL)	Cefalexin	92
Kefzol® (AT, BE, CZ, HR, NL, TR)	Cefazolin	93
Ketek® (AT, BE, DE, ES, FI, FR, GB, HR, IT, NO, PL, PT, SE)	Telithromycin	165
Ketocef® (HR)	Cefuroxime	104
Keimax® (DE)	Ceftibuten	101
Klacid® (AT, CZ, DE, DK, ES, FI, HR, IT, NL, NO,PL, PT, SE, TR)	Clarithromycin	109

Trade Names (Selection)	Generics	Page
Lendacin® (CZ)	Ceftriaxone	102
Lexinor® (FI, SE)	Norfloxacin	145
Logryx® (FR)	Minocycline	141
Lorabid® (AT, GR, NL, SE, TR)	Loracarbef	136
Lorafem® (DE)	Loracarbef	136
Macmiror® (CZ, PL, TR)	Nystatin	146
Macrofuran® (FI)	Nitrofurantoin	145
Maxipime® (AT, BE, CZ, DE, ES, FI, GR, HR, IT, NL, PL, PT, SE, TR)	Cefepime	94
Megacillin oral® (DE)	Penicillin V	151
Merinfec® (AT)	Meropenem	137
Meronem® (BE, CZ, DE, DK, ES, FI, GB, GR, HR, HU, NL, NO, PL, PT, SE, TR)	Meropenem	137
Merrem® (IT)	Meropenem	137
Minocin® (AT, BE, ES, GB, GR, IT, PT)	Minocycline	141
Minocyclin® (DE)	Minocycline	141
Moronal® (DE)	Nystatin	146
Moxacef® (BE, GR, NL)	Cefadroxil	91
Myambutol® (AT, BE, DE, DK, ES, GB, GR, FR, NL)	Ethambutol	121
Mycamine® (DE, IT)	Micafungin	140

Trade Names (Selection)	Generics	Page
Mycobutin® (AT, BE, CZ, DE, GB, GR, IT, NL, PT, TR)	Rifabutin	158
Mycostatin® (AT, BE, DK, ES, FI, FR, GR, IT, NO, PT, SE)	Nystatin	146
Nebcin® (HR, TR)	Tobramycin	168
Nebcina® (DK, FI, NO, SE)	Tobramycin	168
Nebcine® (FR)	Tobramycin	168
Netilin® (GB)	Netilmicin	143
Netrocin® (ES)	Netilmicin	143
Netromicina® (PT)	Netilmicin	143
Netromicine® (BE, CZ, FR, HR, NL, PL, TR)	Netilmicin	143
Netromycin® (GR)	Netilmicin	143
Nettacin® (IT)	Netilmicin	143
Netylin® (DK, FI, NO, SE)	Netilmicin	143
Nicozid (IT)	Isoniazid (INH)	132
Nidrazid® (CZ)	Isoniazid (INH)	132
Nifurantin® (DE)	Nitrofurantoin	145
Ninur® (HR)	Nitrofurantoin	145
Noroxin® (ES, FR, GB, IT, NL, PT, TR)	Norfloxacin	145

Trade Names (Selection)	Generics	Page
Noxafil® (AT, DE, DK, ES, FR, GB, IT, NO, SE)	Posaconazole	154
Nystan® (GB)	Nystatin	146
Obracin® (BE)	Tobramycin	168
Oflocin® (IT)	Ofloxacin	147
Omnacilina® (PT)	Penicillin G (Benzylpenicillin)	149
Oracéfal® (FR)	Cefadroxil	91
Oracilline® (FR)	Penicillin V	151
Orelox® (CZ, DE, DK, ES, FR, GB, GR, IT, NL, SE)	Cefpodoxime proxetil	99
Oributol® (FI)	Ethambutol	121
Orivan® (FI)	Vancomycin	169
Oroken® (FR)	Cefixime	96
Orungal® (HU, PL)	Itraconazole	133
Oxacillin® (CZ)	Oxacillin	148
Panoral® (DE)	Cefaclor	90
Pan-Streptomycin® (GR)	Streptomycin	161
Pantaflux® (IT)	Flucloxacillin	122
Penbritin® (BE, HR, NL)	Ampicillin	83
Penicillin Gruenenthal® (DE)	Penicillin G (Benzylpenicillin)	149
Penidural® (GB)	Penicillin G (Benzylpenicillin)	149

Trade Names (Selection)	Generics	Page
Peniroger® (ES)	Penicillin G (Benzylpenicillin)	149
Penstapho® (BE, IT)	Oxacillin	148
Pentacannat® (DE, ES, FI, FR, GB, GR, IT, NO)	Pentainidine Isethionate	215
Phenoxymethylpenicillin® (GB)	Penicillin V	151
Piperacillin® (DE)	Piperacillin	152
Piperilline® (FR)	Piperacillin	152
Piperital® (IT)	Piperacillin	152
Pipraks® (IT, TR)	Piperacillin	152
Pipril® (AT, CZ, ES, FI, GB, GR, HR, PT)	Piperacillin	152
Piraldina® (TR)	Pyrazinamide	156
Piyeloseptyl® (TR)	Nitrofurantoin	145
Primaxin® (GB, GR)	Imipenem/Cilastatin	130
Primbactam® (IT)	Aztreonam	88
Promid® (TR)	Protionamide	155
Pyrafat® (AT, DE)	Pyrazinamide	156
Refobacin® (DE)	Gentamicin	129
Rifadin® (GB, GR, IT, NL, PT, SE, TR)	Rifampicin	159
Rifamazid® (PL)	Isoniazid (INH) + Rifampicin	160
Rifarm® (FI)	Rifampicin	159

Trade Names (Selection)	Generics	Page
Rifater® (AT, ES, DE, FR, GB, IT, PT, TR)	Isoniazid (INH) + Pyrazinamide + Rifampicin	133
Rifinah® (DE, FR, GB, GR, IT, NL, PT, TR)	Isoniazid (INH) + Rifampicin	133, 160
Rimactan® (BE, DK, ES, FR, NO, SE)	Rifampicin	159
Rimactazid® (DK, NO, SE)	Isoniazid (INH) + Rifampicin	160
Rimcure® (NO, SE)	Isoniazid (INH) + Pyrazinamide + Rifampicin	160
Rimifon® (BE, FR, GB)	Isoniazid (INH)	132
Rimstar® (DK, NO, SE)	Ethambutol + Isoniazid (INH) + Pyrazinamide + Rifampicin	160
Rocefalin® (ES)	Ceftriaxone	102
Rocefin® (IT)	Ceftriaxone	102
Rocephalin® (DK, FI, NO, SE)	Ceftriaxone	102
Rocephin® (AT, DE, GB, GR, HR, NL, PL, PT, TR)	Ceftriaxone	102
Rocéphine® (BE, FR)	Ceftriaxone	102
Rovamicina® (IT)	Spiramycin	224
Rovamycine® (AT, BE, CZ, DE, FR, GR, HR, HU)	Spiramycin	224

Trade Names (Selection)	Generics	Page
Roxithromycin® (DE)	Roxythromycin	160
Rulid® (BE, CZ, FR, GR, IT, PL, TR)	Roxythromycin	160
Rulide® (AT, ES, NL, PT)	Roxythromycin	160
Sempera® (DE)	Itraconazole	133
Siraliden® (PL)	Nitrofurantoin	145
Sobelin® (DE)	Clindamycin	110
Spizef® (AT, DE)	Cefotiam	98
Sporanox® (AT, BE, CZ, DK, FR, FI, GB, GR, IT, NO, PT, SE)	Itraconazole	133
Stapenor® (AT)	Oxacillin	148
Staphylex® (DE, FI)	Flucloxacillin	122
Strep-Deva® (TR)	Streptomycin	161
Streptomycin® (DE)	Streptomycin	161
Streptomicina® (IT)	Streptomycin	161
Supracef® (FI)	Cefixime	96
Suprax® (CZ, GB, HU, IT, TR)	Cefixime	96
Sural® (CZ, HU)	Ethambutol	121
Surlid® (DK, FI, SE)	Roxythromycin	160
Synercid® (AT, CZ, DE, ES, FR, GB, IT, PL)	Quinupristin/Dalfopristin	157

Trade Names (Selection)	Generics	Page
Taketiam® (FR)	Cefotiam	98
Targocid® (AT, BE, CZ, DE, DK, ES, FI, FR, GB, GR, HR, NL, NO, PL, SE, TR)	Teicoplanin	164
Targosid® (IT, PT)	Teicoplanin	164
Tarivid® (DE)	Ofloxacin	147
Tavanic® (AT, BE, CZ, DE, ES, FI, FR, GB, GR, HR, IT, NL, PL, PT, SE, TR)	Levofloxacin	134
Tazobac® (DE)	Piperacillin/Tazobactam	153
Tazocel® (ES)	Piperacillin/Tazobactam	153
Tazocilline® (FR)	Piperacillin/Tazobactam	153
Tazocin® (BE, DK, GB, HU, IT, NL, NO, PL, SE, TR)	Piperacillin/Tazobactam	153
Tebeform® (HU)	Protionamide	155
Tebrazid® (BE)	Pyrazinamide	156
Tetracyclin® (DE)	Tetracycline	166
Tetralysal® (AT, BE, CZ, DK, ES, FI, FR, GB, IT, NO, PL, SE)	Tetracycline	166
Tetrarco® (NL)	Tetracycline	166
Tienam® (BE, CZ, DK, ES, FI, FR, HR, IT, NL, NO, PL, PT, SE, TR)	Imipenem/Cilastatin	130

Trade Names (Selection)	Generics	Page
Tierlite® (GR)	Fluconazole	123
Tisamid® (CZ, FI)	Pyrazinamide	156
TOBI® (DE, FR, GB, PL)	Tobramycin	168
Totapen® (FR)	Ampicillin	83
Trevintix® (GB)	Protionamide	155
Tricef® (SE)	Cefixime	96
Triflucan® (FR, TR)	Fluconazole	123
Tubocin® (HU)	Rifampicin	159
Tygacil® (AT, CZ, DE, ES, FR, GB, IT, NO, SE)	Tigecycline	167
Unacid® (DE, PT)	Ampicillin/Sulbactam	84
Unacim® (FR)	Ampicillin/Sulbactam	84
Unasyn® (AT, CZ, DE, ES, GB, IT, PL)	Ampicillin/Sulbactam	84
Vancocin® (AT, BE, GB, NL, PL, SE, TR)	Vancomycin	169
Vancocina® (IT)	Vancomycin	169
Vfend® (AT, BE, DE, CZ, DK, ES, FI, GB, IT, NL, NO, PL, PT, SE)	Voriconazole	171
Vibativ® (marketing application submitted)	Telavancin	268
Vibramycin® (AT, CZ, DK, GB, GR, HR, NO, NL, SE)	Doxycycline	117

Trade Names (Selection)	Generics	Page
Zienam® (AT, DE)	Imipenem/Cilastatin	130
Zinacef® (BE, CZ, DE, DK, FI, GB, GR, NL, NO, PL, SE, TR)	Cefuroxime	104
Zinnat® (AT, BE, CZ, DK, ES, FI, FR, GB, HR, HU, IT, NL, PL, SE, TR)	Cefuroxime axetil	105
Zithromax® (AT,BE, DE, ES, FI, FR, GB, GR, NL, PT)	Azithromycin	87
Zitromax® (DK, IT, TR)	Azithromycin	87
Zoroxin® (AT, BE, DK)	Norfloxacin	145
Zyvox® (GB)	Linezolid	135
Zyvoxid® (AT, BE, CZ, DE, DK, ES, FI, FR, IT, NL, NO, PL, PT, SE)	Linezolid	135

3 Principles of Antibiotic Therapy

- An antibiotic is not an antipyretic. Raised temperature alone is not an indication for administration of antibiotics.
- Before any antibiotic therapy, attempt to isolate the pathogen.
- If antibiotic therapy shows no effect after 3–4 days, consider the following possibilities: incorrect choice of substance; drug not reaching site of infection; incorrect identification of pathogen (viruses! yeasts!); abscess; defective immune system; drug fever; intravenous catheter; bladder catheter; other foreign bodies (▶ Chap. 13).
- If antibiotic therapy is unnecessary, discontinue it immediately. The longer antibiotics are given, the greater is the danger of selection of resistant bacteria, side effects, and toxicity.
- Most local antibiotics can be replaced by antiseptics (▶ Chap. 20).
- In pyrexia of unknown origin, blood must be taken for culture. A negative result is just as important as a positive one, showing that very probably no sepsis is present.
- If there is any suspicion of systemic infection (even without fever), blood must be cultured and the patient must be kept in hospital for observation.
- Perioperative antibiotic prophylaxis should be as brief as possible. For most operations a single dose is sufficient (▶ Chap. 21).
- "Susceptible" in the antibiogram does not necessarily mean that the substance will be effective. Up to 20% of results are false positive or false negative (methodological deficiencies). Many bacteriological laboratories do not use standardised methods.
- Correct sampling and transport (transport media for throat swabs, wound swabs etc.) are essential for correct diagnosis and thus correct antibiotic therapy (▶ Chap. 5).

- A microscopic sample (pus, CSF, urine etc.) often yields extremely useful pointers to identity of the pathogen 1–3 days before the final bacteriological result.
- Antibiotics are often given for longer than necessary. In most diseases, 3–5 days after cessation of fever suffices.
- Don't change antibiotics too soon! Even the best antibiotic combinations take 2–3 days to bring temperature down to normal.
- Stick to the antibiotics that have served you well in the past. The newest – often most expensive – preparations are usually advantageous only in a few special indications and frequently patchy in their effect on classical infective pathogens. Don't let the most eloquent company representative or the glossiest brochures divert you from your own good clinical or practical experience with standard antibiotics (e.g. penicillin, cotrimoxazole, erythromycin, tetracyclines).
- Exclude allergies before starting antibiotic therapy! Many so-called penicillin allergies reported by patients are not allergies at all, so in the case of doubt run a test.
- Pay attention to possible interactions with other simultaneously administered drugs (▶ Chap. 22).
- For adequate antibiotic therapy, attention must be paid to the situation at the site of infection, for example acidic pH or anaerobic milieu (e.g. abscesses). Aminoglycosides, for instance, have no effect in acidic pH and under anaerobic conditions.
- When administering antibiotics with a narrow therapeutic spectrum (e.g. aminoglycosides, vancomycin), serum levels must be monitored. Peak: max. 30 min after injection or infusion; trough: immediately before the next antibiotic dose.
- Continuous infusion of vancomycin has been demonstrated to reduce nephrotoxic side effects but its impact on the outcome is still under investigations. Studies are ongoing to demonstrate advantages for continuous infusion of piperacillin/tazobactam and meropenem.
- **Single-dose administration of aminoglycosides.** The total dose can be given all at once (infusion over a time of 1 h in 100 ml 0.9% NaCl). Determination of the peak level is no

longer necessary. Following the first or second dose, the trough level is measured immediately before the next dose. It should be <1 mg/l, in no event >2 mg/l (for amikacin >10 mg/l) (beware cumulative effect!). The administration of aminoglycosides in one single daily dose is not recommended in pregnancy or in ascites, meningitis, osteomyelitis, burns or decreased renal function (creatinine clearance <60 mg/l). For children, the data are still too sparse for standard recommendations to be given. Single daily dosing seems appropriate in combination treatment of Gram-negative sepsis and mucoviscidosis. Otherwise, the same contraindications pertain as in adults.

| Antibiotic | Target values (mg/l) | |
	Peak level	Trough level
Gentamicin	5–10	<2
Tobramycin	5–10	<2
Netilmicin	5–10	<2
Amikacin	20–30	<10
Vancomycin	20–50	5–10

Blood culture diagnosis:
- Suspicion of systemic and/or local infections (sepsis, meningitis, osteomyelitis, pneumonia, postoperative infections etc.) or pyrexia of unknown origin: one sample (for aerobic and anaerobic culture) from the first vein, one sample (for aerobic and anaerobic culture) from the second vein.
- Suspicion of bacterial endocarditis: three samples (for aerobic and anaerobic culture) from three different veins (within 3 h).
- Suspicion of intravenous catheter infection: one Isolator® sample (for quantitative culture) from the intravenous catheter; one Isolator® sample and one sample for aerobic culture from a peripheral vein.

Important:
Ensure painstaking skin disinfection; follow the advice of the manufacturer of the blood culture system with regard to the amount of blood to be drawn; document the site and method of sampling.

4 The Most Common Errors in Antibiotic Therapy

- Use of a broad-spectrum antibiotic when a narrow-spectrum agent would suffice
- Excessive duration of therapy
- Intravenous therapy when oral therapy would be equally effective
- Combination therapy when a single antibiotic would suffice
- Failure to change antibiotics when the antibiograms become available
- Failure to adjust the dosage in the case of decreased hepatic or renal function
- Outdated knowledge of antibiotic resistance and thus initial prescription of the wrong agent
- Assuming the worst case, i.e. routinely starting with single or combined antibiotics appropriate for pathogens such as *Pseudomonas* or methicillin-resistant staphylococci

5 Important Infections and Their Microbiological Diagnosis

Infection	Microbiological Diagnosis
Purulent tonsillitis	Throat swab without transport medium (only investigation for group A streptococci)
Meningism	CSF puncture
Pyrexia of unknown origin (always!)	Blood cultures
Foul-smelling infection (e.g. sputum, pus, ascites)	Suspicion of anaerobic infection (special transport media!, pus if possible, do not investigate any swabs)
Purulent wound infection	Pus if possible, wound swabs only from deep tissue
Intravenous catheter infection	Quantitative blood culture (e.g. Isolator®) from IV catheter and also from a peripheral vein (bacteria count at least 5–10 times higher than in IV catheter points to catheter infection); after catheter removal, catheter tip and blood culture
Nosocomial diarrhoea, common after antibiotic therapy	Toxin detection and stool culture for *Clostridium difficile*
Peritonitis with ascites	Pus in special transport medium (anaerobics!) much better than swabs

Infection	Microbiological Diagnosis
Chronic bronchitis with dry cough	Serology for atypical causes of pneumonia (e.g. mycoplasmas, chlamydiae)
Atypical pneumonia in immunodeficient patients	Serology for legionellae, detection of Legionella urinary antigen
Osteomyelitis	Pus, intraoperative material (aspirate) much better than swabs
Secretion or pus from drains	Secretion or pus in transport medium, no drain swabs (frequent secondary contamination)

Basic principles:
- Swift transport of material to the laboratory
- Sampling before the commencement of antibiotic therapy
- If swift transport to the laboratory is impossible, store as follows:

  Room temperature, max. 2–3 h (susceptible species of bacteria may die at 4 °C):
  - Blood cultures
  - Aspirate/puncture fluid from normally sterile body fluids
  - Cerebrospinal fluid
  - Pus, (wound) secretions
  - Biopsy specimens/tissue samples in 0.9% NaCl solution
  - Swabs and catheter tips in transport medium

  Refrigerator at 4 °C, max. 12–24 h:
  - Investigation material with accompanying flora (e.g. sputum, bronchial secretion, stool)
  - Material in which the bacteria count is important (e.g. urine, BAL)
  - Serum for serological investigation (no whole blood, if possible)

6 Cooperation with Microbiologists

- Choose as your partner a microbiologist who will let you know about important results (e.g. α-streptococci in a throat swab, findings of microscopy of samples of pus, joint puncture fluid etc., positive blood cultures) by fax or telephone and not make you wait for the original written report.
- Try to find a microbiologist who will organise the collection and delivery of specimens for you. Long transport times always make for worse bacteriological results.
- Bring the microbiologist to the bedside. A microbiology institute that cannot deliver an infectiology service to the bedside is training theoretical microbiologists, not medical microbiologists. Surgeons and internists are also rarely able to provide a diagnosis by telephone.
- Avoid private "factory labs" even if they are cheaper, unless they are in your neighbourhood and you know someone there who will provide high-quality individual advice and will come to you at the bedside.
- Avoid microbiologists who give you an antibiogram for every isolated bacterium. This is unnecessary work and constitutes profiteering. Many clinical materials are contaminated by bacteria that plainly do not come into question as pathogens. Antibiograms of these microorganisms are usually unnecessary and senseless, e.g. for pneumococci, group A streptococci, blue-green streptococci, *Haemophilus influenzae* (only β-lactamase testing), anaerobes, and meningococci. With the exception of flucytosine (blastomycetes), most antibiograms of fungi are incorrect, because the diameter of the inhibition zone cannot be correlated with the in vitro susceptibility of the blastomycetes.
- Fill in the microbiology request form as accurately and specifically as possible; explain precisely what you want. For instance, don't simply write "throat swab – pathogenic microorganisms – antibiogram". Rather, word your request as spe-

cifically as possible, e.g. "throat swab – β-haemolytic group A streptococci – no antibiogram". This holds for stool samples too. Don't just write "stool – pathogenic microorganisms – antibiogram", but, for example, "rotaviruses, salmonellae, shigellae" if an infant or small child is involved, or "salmonellae and *Campylobacter*" for adults, in whom rotaviruses are practically never found.

• Ask your microbiologist to give you at least half-yearly updates on the resistance displayed by the five or six pathogens most commonly encountered in your specialty – without "copy strains", i.e. the same pathogen from the same patient.

• Please adhere strictly to your microbiologist's recommendations regarding isolation and transport of the material for examination. For instance, you cannot expect to receive useful information if you send a sample of urine that has been standing around for several hours at room temperature. If you send the tip of a bladder catheter or bladder drain, rather than urine or drainage fluid, the microbiologist will often isolate contaminating bacteria, not those responsible for infection.

7 Resistance of Major Clinical Pathogens

Table 7.1 shows the susceptibility or resistance displayed in vitro by the major clinical pathogens (+ = susceptible; ± = intermediate; 0 = resistant). In vitro susceptibility to a particular antibiotic does not automatically mean efficacy of that agent in vivo.

Tab. 7.1 Resistance of major clinical pathogens

	Acinetobacter	Aeromonas	Actinomyces	Bacteroides fragilis	Burkholderia cepacia	Chlamydiae	Citrobacter	Clostridia	Corynebacterium jekeium	Enterobacter	Enterococcus faecalis	Enterococcus faecium	Escherichia coli
Amikacin	0	0	0	0	0	0	±	0	0	+	0	0	+
Amoxicillin, ampicillin	0	0	+	0	0	0	±	+	0	0	+	0	+
Amoxicillin/clavulanate	0	+	+	+	0	0	0	+	0	0	+	0	+
Ampicillin/sulbactam	+	+	+	+	0	0	0	+	0	0	+	0	+
Azithromycin	0	0	+	0	0	+	0	+	0	0	0	0	0
Aztreonam	0	+	0	0	0	0	+	0	0	+	0	0	+
Cefaclor	0	±	0	0	0	0	±	±	0	0	0	0	+
Cefadroxil	0	±	0	0	0	0	0	+	0	0	0	0	+
Cefalexin	0	±	0	0	0	0	0	+	0	0	0	0	+
Cefazolin	0	0	0	0	0	0	0	+	0	0	0	0	+
Cefepime	±	+	0	0	±	0	+	+	0	+	0	0	+
Cefixime	0	+	0	0	0	0	+	0	0	±	0	0	+
Cefotaxime	+	+	0	0	+	0	+	+	0	+	0	0	+
Cefotiam	0	+	0	0	0	0	±	+	0	±	0	0	+
Cefoxitin	0	±	0	+	0	0	±	+	0	0	0	0	+

Haemophilus influenzae	Klebsiellae	Legionellae	Listeria monocytogenes	Moraxella catarrhalis	Mycoplasma pneumoniae	Proteus mirabilis	Proteus vulgaris	Providencia	Pseudomonas aeruginosa	Salmonellae	Serratia	Shigellae	Staphylococcus aureus (MSSA)	Staphylococcus aureus (MRSA)	Staphylococcus epidermidis	Stenotrophomonas maltophilia	Streptococci A, B, C, G	Streptococcus pneumoniae	Streptococcus viridans	Yersinia enterocolitica
+	+	0	+	+	0	+	+	+	+	+	+	+	+	0	±	±	0	0	0	+
±	0	0	+	±	0	+	0	0	0	+	0	+	±	0	+	0	+	+	+	0
+	+	0	+	+	0	+	±	+	0	+	0	+	+	0	+	0	+	+	+	±
+	+	0	+	+	0	+	±	+	0	+	0	+	+	0	+	0	+	+	+	±
+	0	+	+	+	+	0	0	0	0	0	0	0	+	0	±	0	+	+	+	±
+	+	0	0	+	0	+	+	+	+	+	+	+	+	0	0	0	0	0	0	+
±	+	0	0	+	0	+	0	0	0	0	0	0	+	0	±	0	+	+	+	0
0	+	0	0	+	0	+	0	0	0	0	0	0	+	0	±	0	+	+	+	0
0	+	0	0	0	0	+	0	0	0	0	0	0	+	0	±	0	+	+	+	0
+	+	0	0	+	0	+	0	0	0	0	+	0	+	0	±	0	+	+	+	0
+	+	0	0	+	0	+	+	+	+	+	+	+	+	0	±	0	+	+	+	+
+	+	0	0	+	0	+	+	+	0	+	±	0	+	0	0	0	+	+	+	+
+	+	0	0	+	0	+	+	+	±	+	+	+	+	0	±	0	+	+	+	+
+	+	0	0	+	0	+	+	±	+	0	+	+	+	0	±	0	+	+	+	±
+	+	0	0	+	0	+	+	+	0	+	0	+	+	0	±	0	+	+	+	±

Tab. 7.1 (continued)

	Acinetobacter	Aeromonas	Actinomyces	Bacteroides fragilis	Burkholderia cepacia	Chlamydiae	Citrobacter	Clostridia	Corynebacterium jekeium	Enterobacter	Enterococcus faecalis	Enterococcus faecium	Escherichia coli
Cefpodoxime proxetil	0	+	0	0	0	0	+	+	0	0	0	0	+
Ceftazidime	+	+	0	0	+	0	±	+	0	+	0	0	+
Ceftibuten	0	+	0	0	+	0	+	+	0	±	0	0	+
Ceftriaxone	+	+	0	0	+	0	+	+	0	+	0	0	+
Cefuroxime	0	+	0	0	0	0	±	+	0	±	0	0	+
Chloramphenicol	0	+	+	+	+	+	+	0	+	0	0	0	+
Ciprofloxacin	+	+	0	0	0	±	+	±	+	+	±	0	+
Clarithromycin	0	0	+	0	0	+	0	+	0	0	±	±	0
Clindamycin	0	0	+	+	0	+	0	0	0	0	0	0	0
Cotrimoxazole	0	+	+	0	+	±	0	+	0	0	±	0	+
Daptomycin	0	0	0	0	0	0	0	±	+	0	+	+	0
Doxycycline	0	+	+	±	0	+	0	+	0	0	0	0	±
Ertapenem	0	0	+	+	0	0	+	±	0	+	0	0	+
Erythromycin	0	0	+	0	0	+	0	±	±	0	0	0	0
Flucloxacillin	0	0	0	0	0	0	0	0	0	0	0	0	0
Gentamicin	0	0	0	0	0	0	±	0	0	+	0	0	+
Imipenem	+	+	+	+	+	0	+	+	0	+	+	±	+
Levofloxacin	+	+	+	+	±	+	+	±	+	+	+	0	+
Linezolid	0	0	0	±	0	0	0	+	+	0	+	+	0
Loracarbef	0	±	0	0	0	0	±	0	0	0	0	0	+
Meropenem	+	+	+	+	+	0	+	+	0	+	±	0	+
Metronidazole	0	0	±	+	0	0	0	+	0	0	0	0	0
Mezlocillin	0	+	+	+	+	0	+	+	0	+	+	±	+
Moxifloxacin	+	+	0	+	0	+	+	±	+	+	±	0	+
Netilmicin	0	0	0	0	0	0	±	0	0	+	0	0	+
Nitrofurantoin	0	+	0	0	0	0	+	0	0	±	±	0	+

Haemophilus influenzae	Klebsiellae	Legionellae	Listeria monocytogenes	Moraxella catarrhalis	Mycoplasma pneumoniae	Proteus mirabilis	Proteus vulgaris	Providencia	Pseudomonas aeruginosa	Salmonellae	Serratia	Shigellae	Staphylococcus aureus (MSSA)	Staphylococcus aureus (MRSA)	Staphylococcus epidermidis	Stenotrophomonas maltophilia	Streptococci A, B, C, G	Streptococcus pneumoniae	Streptococcus viridans	Yersinia enterocolitica
+	+	0	0	+	0	+	±	+	0	+	0	+	+	0	±	0	+	+	+	+
+	+	0	0	+	0	+	+	+	+	+	+	+	+	0	±	±	+	+	+	±
+	+	0	0	+	0	+	+	+	0	+	±	+	0	0	0	0	+	±	0	+
+	+	0	0	+	0	+	+	+	±	+	+	+	+	0	±	0	+	+	+	+
+	+	0	0	+	0	+	0	+	0	+	0	+	+	0	±	0	+	+	+	±
+	±	0	±	+	+	±	±	±	0	+	0	+	±	0	0	+	+	+	+	+
+	+	+	±	+	+	+	+	+	+	+	+	+	+	0	±	+	±	±	±	±
+	0	+	+	+	+	0	0	0	0	0	0	0	+	0	+	0	+	0	+	0
0	0	0	±	0	0	0	0	0	0	0	0	0	+	0	0	0	+	+	+	0
+	0	+	+	+	0	+	0	+	0	+	±	+	+	0	±	+	+	+	0	+
0	0	0	0	0	0	0	0	0	0	0	0	0	+	+	+	0	+	+	+	0
+	0	+	+	+	+	0	0	0	0	±	0	±	±	0	0	0	±	+	+	+
+	+	0	+	+	0	+	+	+	0	+	+	+	+	0	±	0	+	+	+	+
±	0	+	+	+	+	0	0	0	0	0	0	0	±	0	±	0	+	+	+	0
0	0	0	0	0	0	0	0	0	0	0	0	0	+	0	±	0	+	+	+	0
+	±	0	0	+	0	+	±	±	±	+	±	+	+	±	±	0	+	+	+	+
+	+	+	+	+	0	+	+	+	+	+	+	+	+	0	+	0	+	+	+	+
+	+	+	±	+	+	+	+	+	+	+	+	+	+	0	+	±	+	+	±	+
±	0	+	±	±	+	0	0	0	0	0	0	0	+	+	+	0	+	+	+	0
+	+	0	0	+	0	+	0	0	0	0	0	0	+	0	±	0	+	+	+	0
+	+	+	+	+	0	+	+	+	+	+	+	+	0	+	0	+	+	+	+	+
0	0	0	0	0	0	0	0	0	0	0	0	0	0	0	0	0	0	0	0	0
+	+	0	+	0	0	+	+	+	±	+	+	+	0	0	0	0	+	+	+	+
+	+	+	+	+	+	+	+	+	0	+	±	+	+	0	+	+	+	+	+	+
+	+	0	+	+	0	+	+	+	+	+	+	+	0	±	0	0	0	0	0	+
+	±	0	0	0	0	+	0	0	0	+	0	0	+	0	+	0	+	+	+	0

Tab. 7.1 (continued)

	Acinetobacter	Aeromonas	Actinomyces	Bacteroides fragilis	Burkholderia cepacia	Chlamydiae	Citrobacter	Clostridia	Corynebacterium jekeium	Enterobacter	Enterococcus faecalis	Enterococcus faecium	Escherichia coli
Norfloxacin	0	+	0	0	0	0	+	0	0	+	0	0	+
Ofloxacin	±	+	±	0	0	+	+	±	+	+	±	0	+
Penicillin	0	0	+	0	0	0	0	+	0	0	0	0	+
Piperacillin	0	+	+	±	±	0	+	+	0	+	+	±	+
Piperacillin/tazobactam[1]	+	+	+	+	±	0	+	+	0	+	+	±	+
Quinupristin/dalfopristin	0	0	+	0	0	+	0	+	+	0	0	+	0
Roxithromycin	0	0	+	0	0	+	0	+	0	0	±	±	0
Telithromycin	0	0	+	±	0	+	0	+	0	0	±	±	0
Tigecycline	+	+	+	+	+	+	+	+	+	+	+	+	+
Tobramycin	+	0	0	0	0	0	0	0	0	+	0	0	+
Vancomycin/teicoplanin	0	0	+	0	0	0	0	+	+	0	+	±	0

[1] Or piperacillin/sulbactam

Haemophilus influenzae	Klebsiellae	Legionellae	Listeria monocytogenes	Moraxella catarrhalis	Mycoplasma pneumoniae	Proteus mirabilis	Proteus vulgaris	Providencia	Pseudomonas aeruginosa	Salmonellae	Serratia	Shigellae	Staphylococcus aureus (MSSA)	Staphylococcus aureus (MRSA)	Staphylococcus epidermidis	Stenotrophomonas maltophilia	Streptococci A, B, C, G	Streptococcus pneumoniae	Streptococcus viridans	Yersinia enterocolitica
+	+	+	0	+	0	+	+	+	±	+	+	+	±	0	±	0	0	0	0	+
+	+	+	±	+	+	+	+	+	±	+	+	+	+	0	+	±	±	±	±	+
±	0	0	+	0	0	+	0	0	0	±	0	0	0	0	0	0	+	+	+	0
+	±	0	+	±	0	+	+	+	+	+	±	+	±	0	±	±	+	+	+	+
+	+	0	+	+	0	+	+	+	+	+	+	+	+	0	+	±	+	+	+	+
±	0	+	+	+	+	0	0	0	0	0	0	+	+	+	0	+	+	+	+	0
+	0	+	+	+	+	0	0	0	0	0	0	+	0	+	0	+	+	+	+	0
+	0	+	+	+	+	0	0	0	0	0	0	+	0	0	0	+	+	+	+	0
+	+	0	+	+	0	+	+	+	+	+	+	+	+	0	±	0	0	0	0	+
0	0	0	+	0	0	0	0	0	0	0	0	0	+	+	+	0	+	+	+	0

The European Antimicrobial Resistance Surveillance Network (EARS-NET, formerly EARSS) provides reference data on antimicrobial resistance in European nations and is coordinated and funded by the Euroean Centre for Disease Prevention and Control (ECDC). The EARS data can be found on the website: http://www.ecdc.europa.eu/en/activities/surveillance/EARS-Net

The resistance pattern can vary within a hospital complex, even from ward to ward. Therefore, knowledge of the local resistance situation is important.

The following figures provide an overview of the EARSS data in 2008.

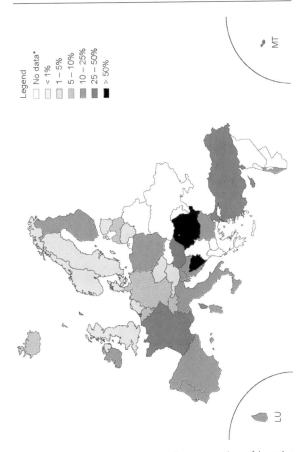

Abb. 7.1 *Streptococcus pneumoniae:* proportion of invasive isolates nonsusceptible to penicillin (PNSP) in 2008. © EARSS

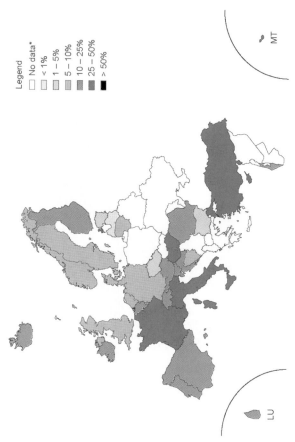

Abb. 7.2 *Streptococcus pneumoniae:* proportion of invasive isolates resistant to erythromycin in 2008. © EARSS

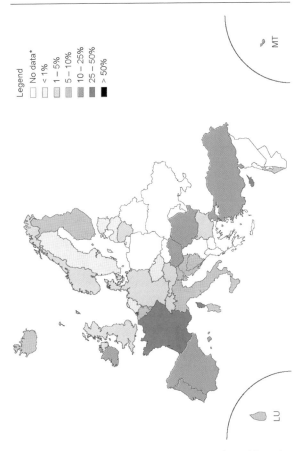

Abb. 7.3 *Streptococcus pneumoniae:* proportion of invasive isolates with dual resistance to erythromycin and penicillin in 2008. © EARSS

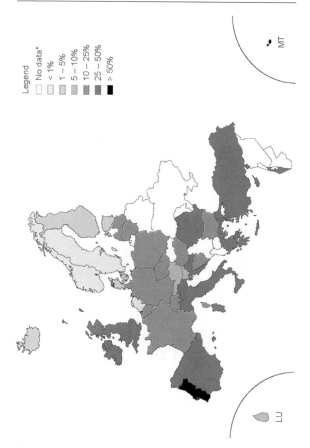

Abb. 7.4 *Staphylococcus aureus:* proportion of invasive isolates resistant to oxacillin (MRSA) in 2008. © EARSS

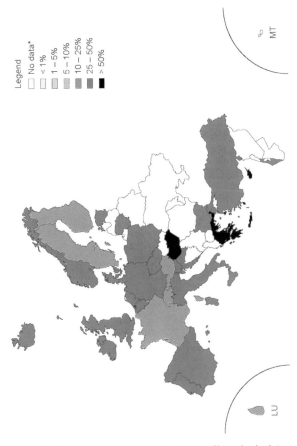

Abb. 7.5 *Enterococcus faecalis:* proportion of invasive isolates with high-level resistance to aminoglycosides in 2008.
© EARSS

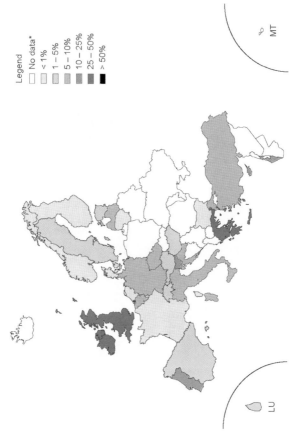

Abb. 7.6 *Enterococcus faecium:* proportion of invasive isolates resistant to vancomycin in 2008. © EARSS

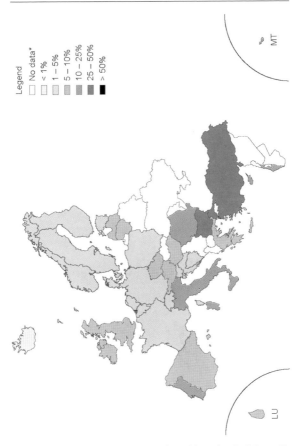

Abb. 7.7 *Escherichia coli:* proportion of invasive isolates with resistance to third-generation cephalosporins in 2008.
© EARSS

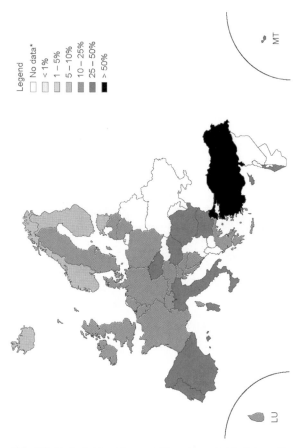

Abb. 7.8 *Escherichia coli:* proportion of invasive isolates with resistance to fluoroquinolones in 2008. © EARSS

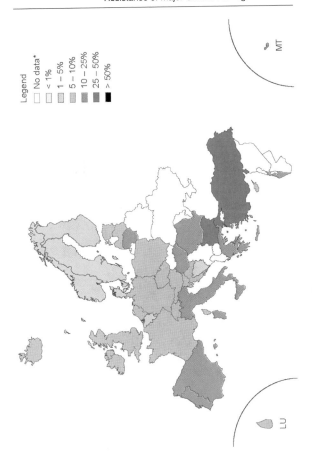

Abb. 7.9 *Escherichia coli:* proportion of invasive isolates with resistance to aminoglycosides in 2008. © EARSS

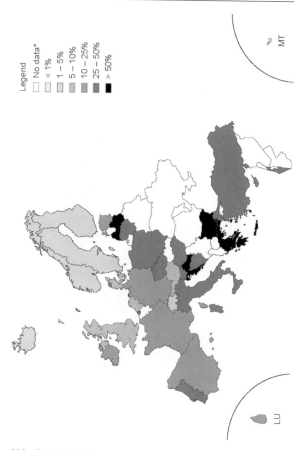

Abb. 7.10 *Klebsiella pneumoniae:* proportion of invasive isolates resistant to third-generation cephalosporins in 2008.
© EARSS

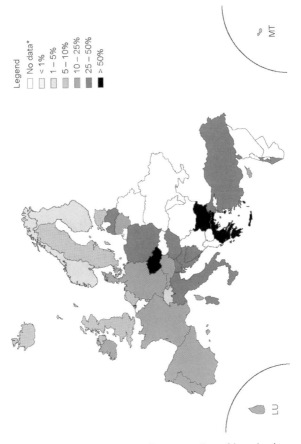

Abb. 7.11 *Klebsiella pneumoniae:* proportion of invasive isolates resistant to fluoroquinolones in 2008. © EARSS

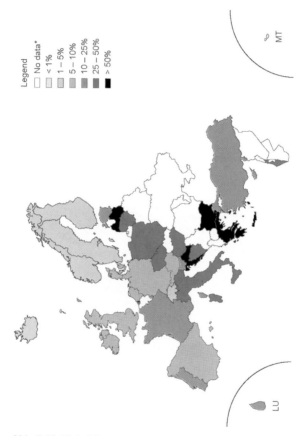

Abb. 7.12 *Klebsiella pneumoniae:* proportion of invasive isolates resistant to aminoglycosides in 2008. © EARSS

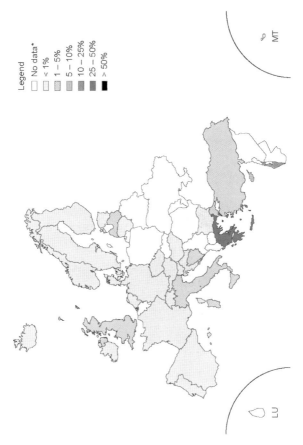

Abb. 7.13 *Klebsiella pneumoniae:* proportion of invasive isolates resistant to carbapenems in 2008. © EARSS

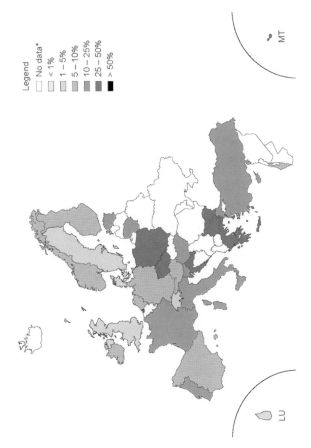

Abb. 7.14 *Pseudomonas aeruginosa:* proportion of invasive isolates resistant to piperacillins in 2008. © EARSS

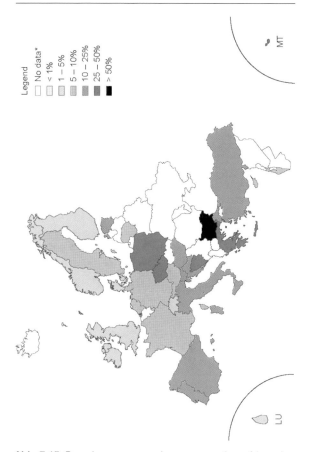

Abb. 7.15 *Pseudomonas aeruginosa:* proportion of invasive isolates resistant to ceftazidime in 2008. © EARSS

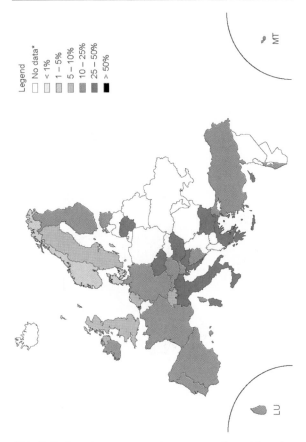

Abb. 7.16 *Pseudomonas aeruginosa:* proportion of invasive isolates resistant to fluoroquinolones in 2008. © EARSS

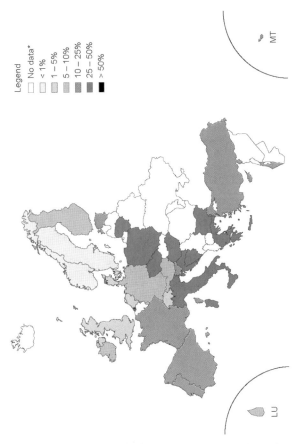

Abb. 7.17 *Pseudomonas aeruginosa:* proportion of invasive isolates resistant to aminoglycosides in 2008. © EARSS

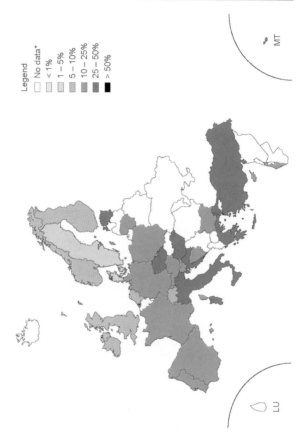

Abb. 7.18 *Pseudomonas aeruginosa:* proportion of invasive isolates resistant to carbapenems in 2008. © EARSS

8 The Most Frequent Pathogens – Choice of Antibiotics

Tab. 8.1 The most frequent pathogens – choice of antibiotics

Pathogen	First choice[1]	Alternatives
Acinetobacter baumannii	Carbapenems	Ampicillin/sulbactam, cotrimoxazole, colistin (MDR), quinolones, ± aminoglycosides, tigecycline
Actinomyces israelii	Penicillin G, ampicillin	Doxycyclines, ceftriaxone
Aeromonas hydrophila	Quinolones	Cotrimoxazole, cephalosporins (3rd/4th gen.)
Alcaligenes xylosoxidans	Carbapenems	Cotrimoxazole, AP-penicillins
Aspergillus species	Voriconazole	Caspofungin, amphotericin B, micafungin, posaconazole, itraconazole
Bacillus anthracis	Ciprofloxacin, levofloxacin	Doxycycline + clindamycin or rifampin
Bacillus cereus, B. subtilis	Vancomycin, clindamycin	Carbapenems, quinolones
Bacteroides fragilis	Metronidazole	Piperacillin/tazobactam, ampicillin/sulbactam, amoxicillin/clavulanate
Bartonellae	Macrolides, quinolones	Doxycyclines

Tab. 8.1 (continued)

Pathogen	First choice[1]	Alternatives
Bordetella species	Macrolides	Cotrimoxazole
Borrelia burgdorferi	Penicillin, doxy-cycline, ceftriax-one, amoxicillin	Cefuroxime axetil, cefpodoxime proxetil, macrolides
Brucellae	Doxycycline + rifampicin, doxy-cycline + gen-tamicin, doxycy-cline + strepto-mycin	Cotrimoxazole + gentamicin
Burkholderia cepacia	Cotrimoxazole, ciprofloxacin	Meropenem
Campylobacter species	Macrolides	Tetracyclines, quinolones
Candida species	Fluconazole	Voriconazole, caspo-fungin, anidulafungin, amphotericin B
Chlamydiae	Tetracyclines	Macrolides, quinolones (group III)
Citrobacter species	Carbapenems, cefepime	Quinolones
Clostridium difficile	Metronidazole	Vancomycin
Clostridium species	Penicillin G	Tetracyclines, clindamycin
Corynebacterium diphtheriae	Penicillin G + antitoxin admi-nistration	Macrolides, clindamycin

Tab. 8.1 (continued)

Pathogen	First choice[1]	Alternatives
Corynebacterium jeikeium	Vancomycin, teicoplanin	Penicillin G + aminoglycoside
Coxiella burnetii	Doxycycline	Quinolones, erythromycin
Eikenella corrodens	Penicillin G, ampicillin	Quinolones
Enterobacter species	Carbapenems	Quinolones
Enterococcus faecalis	Ampicillin	Vancomycin, teicoplanin
Enterococcus faecium	Vancomycin, teicoplanin	Quinupristin/dalfopristin, linezolid
Enterococcus faecium (VRE)[2]	Linezolid, tigecycline	Quinupristin/dalfopristin, fosfomycin[3]
Escherichia coli	Cephalosporins (2nd/3rd gen.)	Quinolones, piperacillin/ tazobactam or sulbactam
Flavobacterium meningosepticum	Vancomycin + rifampicin	Cotrimoxazole, rifampicin
Francisella tularensis	Aminoglycosides, doxycycline	Streptomycin, ciprofloxacin
Fusobacteria	Penicillin G	Metronidazole, clindamycin
Gardnerella vaginalis	Metronidazole	Clindamycin
Gonococci	Cephalosporins (2nd/3rd gen.)	Quinolones, spectinomycin

Tab. 8.1 (continued)

Pathogen	First choice[1]	Alternatives
Haemophilus influenzae	Cephalosporins, ampicillin/sulbactam, amoxicillin/clavulanate	Cotrimoxazole, macrolides, quinolones
Helicobacter pylori[3]	Amoxicillin, clarithromycin	Metronidazole, levofloxacin
Kingella kingae	Penicillin G, ampicillin	Cephalosporins, aminoglycosides
Klebsiellae	Cephalosporins (3rd gen.)	Quinolones
Lactobacilli	Penicillin G	Erythromycin
Legionella pneumophila	Azithromycin, quinolones, Carbapems	Macrolides
Leptospirae	Penicillin G	Tetracyclines
Listeriae	Ampicillin ± aminoglycosides	Penicillin G, cotrimoxazole
Meningococci	Penicillin G	Cefotaxime, ceftriaxone
Moraxella catarrhalis	Cotrimoxazole, amoxicillin/clavulanate	Oral cephalosporins (2nd/3rd gen.), macrolides, quinolones
Morganellae	Cephalosporins (3rd gen.)	Quinolones (gr. II, III), carbapenems
Mycoplasma pneumoniae	Macrolides	Tetracyclines, quinolones (gr. III, IV)
Nocardiae	Cotrimoxazole	Minocycline
Pasteurella multocida	Penicillin G	Cephalosporins (2nd/3rd gen.), tetracyclines, cotrimoxazole

Tab. 8.1 (continued)

Pathogen	First choice[1]	Alternatives
Peptostrepto-cocci	Penicillin G	Clindamycin, metronidazole
Pneumococci	Penicillin G	Macrolides, cephalosporins
Pneumococci (penicillin resistant)	Cephalosporins (3rd gen.)	Quinolones (gr. III, IV), vancomycin ± rifampin, telithromycin
Propionibacteria	Penicillin G	Tetracyclines, clindamycin
Proteus mirabilis	Ampicillin/ sulbactam	Cephalosporins, cotrimoxazole
Proteus vulgaris	Cephalosporins (3rd gen.)	Quinolones, aminoglycosides
Providencia species	Cephalosporins (3rd gen.)	Quinolones, cotrimoxazole
Pseudomonas aeruginosa	Piperacillin, AP-cephalosporins[4] both ± aminogly-cosides	Ciprofloxacin, carbapenems
Rickettsiae	Tetracyclines	Quinolones, chloramphenicol
Salmonella typhi/paratyphi	Quinolones, cephalosporins (3rd gen.)	Cotrimoxazole, chloramphenicol
Salmonella enteritidis	Usually no anti-biotic therapy	–
Serratia marcescens	Cephalosporins (3rd gen.), quinolones	Carbapenems, aminoglycosides

Tab. 8.1 (continued)

Pathogen	First choice[1]	Alternatives
Shigellae	Quinolones	Cotrimoxazole, azithromycin
Staphylococci (MSSA)[5]	Oxacillins	Cephalosporins (1st/2nd gen.), clindamycin, vancomycin, teicoplanin
Staphylococci (MRSA)[6]	Vancomycin ± rifampin, teicoplanin	Linezolid, daptomycin, tigecycline, cotrimoxazole
Staphylococci (MRSE)[7]	Vancomycin, teicoplanin ± rifampicin	Daptomycin, tigecycline, quinupristin/dalfopristin
Stenotrophomonas maltophilia	Cotrimoxazole	Quinolones, minocycline
Streptococci (aerobic and anaerobic)	Penicillin G	Cephalosporins, macrolides
Treponema pallidum	Penicillin G	Doxycycline, ceftriaxone
Ureaplasma	Tetracyclines	Macrolides
Vibrio	Tetracyclines	Cotrimoxazole, quinolones
Yersinia enterocolitica	Doxycycline + aminoglycosides	Cotrimoxazole, quinolones

[1] Until antibiogram available
[2] Vancomycin-resistant enterococci
[3] Combination therapy
[4] Antipseudomonal cephalosporins: ceftazidime, cefepime
[5] Methicillin(=oxacillin-)-sensitive *S. aureus*
[6] Methicillin(=oxacillin-)-resistant *S. aureus*
[7] Methicillin(=oxacillin-)-resistant *S. epidermidis*

9 Antibiotics, Antimycotics: Spectrum – Dosage – Adverse Effects – Costs

Amikacin
Amicasil® (GR, IT), Amikacin® (DE), Amikaver® (TR), Amikin® (CZ, GB, HR, HU, PL), Amiklin® (FR), Amukin® (BE, NL), BB K8® (IT), Biclin® (ES, PT), Biklin® (AT, DK, FI, SE)

Spectrum:
Gram-positive (staphylococci; not: pneumococci, streptococci, enterococci) and Gram-negative bacteria, in particular gentamicin-resistant pathogens; only weakly effective against *H. influenzae*; synergy with β-lactam antibiotics against enterobacteria

Dosage:

- Adults   10–15 mg/kg/day divided into 1–3 doses i.m., i.v. preferably 30–60 min brief infusion

- Children >1 year old   15 mg/kg/day i.m., i.v. divided into 1–3 doses; infusion over 1–2 h

- Neonates   initially 10 mg/kg/day i.m., i.v. divided into 1–3 doses, then 15 mg/kg/day i.v., i.m. divided into 2 doses (even at body weight under 1,200 g); infusion over 1–2 h

- Neonates >1 week old   initially 10 mg/kg/day i.v., i.m., then 15 mg/kg/day i.v., i.m. divided into 3 doses, from 4 weeks old single daily dosing possible; infusion over 1–2 h

In renal	CrCl[1]	Max. dose (g)	DI(h)
insufficiency	120	0.25	6
(adults):	45	0.125	8
	18	0.125	12
	8	0.1	12
	2	0.125[2]	24
	0.5	0.125[2]	24–48[3]

[1] Calculation of CrCl according to Crockroft-Gault equation
[2] In life-threatening circumstances initial dose of 0.5 g
[3] Two to three haemodialyses/week are considered necessary in such cases. One normal dose initially

In renal	CrCl	Dose (% of normal dose)
insufficiency	40	40 (divided into 2 doses)
(children):	20	25 (divided into 2 doses); LD 10 mg/kg
	10	20 (divided into 2 doses); LD 7.5 mg/kg
	Anuria	10 (single dose); LD 5 mg/kg or 33% after HD

Adverse effects:
Nephro- and ototoxicity particularly with long duration of therapy (>10 days), high dosage (more than 15 g, peak level >32 µg/ml, trough level >10 µg/ml), previous aminoglycoside therapy and simultaneous administration of furosemide, ethacrynic acid or other nephro- and ototoxic substances. Blood count changes, arthralgia, fever, hypersensitivity reactions, neuromuscular blockade

Contraindications:
Parenteral administration in first 3 months of pregnancy, give from 4th month of pregnancy onward only if patient's life is

endangered; myasthenia gravis; existing kidney or hearing impairment

Remarks:
Aminoglycoside of choice for gentamicin-resistant bacteria and for *Serratia*. Aminoglycoside solutions not to be mixed with penicillins or cephalosporins (deactivation of the aminoglycosides)

Amoxicillin
Actimoxi® (ES), Agram® (FR), Aktil® (HU), Alfoxil® (TR), Almacin® (HR), Almodan® (GB), Amimox® (NO, SE), Amoclen® (CZ), Amorion® (FI), Amotaks® (PL), Amox® (IT), Amoxi® (BE), Amoxillin® (NO), Amoxypen® (DE)

Spectrum:
Gram-positive (not *S. aureus*) and Gram-negative bacteria (*H. influenzae*: ca. 10% resistance)

Dosage:

• Adults	1.5–3 g (max. 4–6 g)/day divided into 3–4 doses
• Children older than 3 months <40 kg	25–45 mg/kg/day divided into 3–4 doses
In renal insufficiency (adults):	If CrCl <30 ml/min, reduction to $^2/_3$ of normal dose; if CrCl <20 ml/min, to $^1/_3$ of normal dose

In renal insufficiency (children):	CrCl	Dose (% of normal dose)
	40	100
	20	60 (divided into 2 doses)
	10	30 (divided into 2 doses)
	Anuria	15 (single dose) or 30 after HD

Adverse effects:
Gastrointestinal symptoms, diarrhoea, exanthema (on average 8%, especially in patients with infectious mononucleosis and other viral diseases, lymphocytic leukaemia), fever, rarely increased transaminases, interstitial nephritis

Contraindications:
Penicillin allergy, infectious mononucleosis and chronic lymphocytic leukaemia (in >50% of exanthemas)

Remarks:
Two to three times more efficiently resorbed than ampicillin

Amoxicillin/Clavulanate
Abba® (IT), Aktil® (HU), Amiclav® (GB), Amoclan® (AT, NL), Amoclavam® (PT), Amoklavin® (TR), Amoxi comp® (FI), Augmentan® (DE), Augmentin® (BE, CZ, PL), Clamoxyl® (ES)

Spectrum:
Gram-positive (not *E. faecium*) and Gram-negative bacteria, particularly *H. influenzae*, ß-lactamase forming pathogens, anaerobes

Dosage:

- Adults and children >12 years — 625–1,250 mg (tablet) p.o. q8h or 1,000 mg (film tablet) p.o. q12h; 1.2–2.2 g i.v. q8h

- Children >1 year old — 20–40 mg/kg/day p.o. divided into 3 doses; in otitis media 90 mg/kg/day i.v. divided into 3 doses

- Infants >3 months old — 60–96 mg/kg/day i.v. divided into 2–3 doses; 30–50 mg/kg/day p.o. divided into 3 doses

In renal insufficiency (adults):	With CrCl of 30–10 ml/min, initially 1.2 g i.v. q24h, then 600 mg i.v. q12h; with CrCl <10 ml/min, initially 1.2 g i.v., then 600 mg i.v. q24h. With haemodialysis, initially 1.2 g i.v., at end of haemodialysis additionally 600 mg i.v.

In renal insufficiency (children):

CrCl	Dose (% of normal dose)
40	100
20	25 (divided into 2 doses)
10	25 (divided into 2 doses)
Anuria	15 (single dose) or 30 after HD

Adverse effects:
Gastrointestinal symptoms, diarrhoea, exanthema (on average 1–2%; more frequent in patients with infectious mononucleosis, other viral diseases, or lymphocytic leukaemia), fever, rarely increased transaminases, interstitial nephritis; positive Coombs test, hepatitis/cholestatic jaundice (very rare)

Contraindications:
Penicillin allergy, infectious mononucleosis and lymphocytic leukaemia (exanthema), severe liver function impairment; use in pregnancy only after painstaking benefit-risk analysis

---

Amphotericin B
Amphocycline® (FR), Ampho-Moronal® (AT, DE), Amphotericin B® (DE), Fungilin® (DK, GB), Fungizona® (ES), Fungizone® (FI, NL, IT, NO, SE)

Spectrum:
Effective against many *Candida* species, aspergilli, histoplasmosis, sporotrichosis, cryptococcosis, blastomycosis etc.; not against dermatophytes

Dosage:

• Adults and children Amphotericin B	Initial dose of 0.1–0.25 mg/kg/day i.v., increase incrementally by 0.1–0.25 mg/kg daily to a total daily dosage of 0.6–1 mg/kg/day i.v.; in life-threatening infection begin with 0.5–0.7 (max. 1) mg/kg/day i.v., also in combination with 5-flucytosine (5-FC). Combination with flucytosine: day 1: 100–150 mg/kg/day flucytosine + 0.1 mg/kg/day amphotericin B, day 2: 150 mg/kg/day flucytosine + 0.2 mg/kg/day amphotericin B, day 3 onward: 150 mg/kg/day flucytosine + 0.3 mg/kg/day amphotericin B. Test sensitivity to flucytosine!
• Liposomal amphotericin	3-5 mg/kg/day i.v.
• Lipid-based amphotericin	5 mg/kg/day i.v.
In renal insufficiency (adults and children):	Administration of amphotericin B does not lead to accumulation, even in patients with total renal insufficiency

Adverse effects:
Fever, chills (amphotericin B > liposomal > lipid-based) vomiting, thrombophlebitis, nephrotoxicity (with haematuria, proteinuria, azotaemia, hyperkaliuria, hypokalaemia etc.), blood count alterations, hepatotoxicity, peripheral and central neurotoxicity, back pain (with liposomal amphotericin B)

Contraindications:
Threatened renal failure and combination with other nephrotoxic medications, severe liver function impairment (but no

dose adjustment necessary with liposomal amphotericin); during pregnancy and lactation only if patient's life is endangered

Remarks:
Continuous monitoring of renal function and serum electrolytes, blood count and liver function necessary; compensation of hyponatraemia lessens the nephrotoxicity; addition of heparin to infusion lowers the risk of thrombophlebitis; if febrile reaction occurs, give corticosteroids; if signs of kidney damage are noted (serum creatinine >3 mg/dl), interrupt treatment until serum creatinine returns to normal. Continuous infusion of amphotericin B reduces the toxicity and permits administration of up to 2 mg/kg/day.

Ampicillin
Abetathen® (GR), Alongamicina® (ES), Amfipen® (GB), Amplital® (IT), Ampicillin® (DE, HU), Ampicin® (FI), Amplifar® (PT), Binotal® (AT), Doktacilin® (DK, NO, SE), Fortapen® (BE), Penbritin® (BE, HR, NL), Totapen® (FR)

Spectrum:
As for amoxicillin; agent of choice for *Listeria*

Dosage:

- Adults and children >6 years
  0.5–1 g p.o. q6–8h, 1.5–6 (max. 15) g/day i.v. in 2–4 doses

- Children >1 year old
  50–100 mg/kg/day p.o. divided into 2–4 doses, 100–400 mg/kg/day i.v. divided into 2–4 doses

- Neonates
  25–50 mg/kg/day p.o. divided into 2–4 doses (body weight under 1,200 g: 25–50 mg/kg/day divided into 2–4 doses), 50 mg/kg/day i.m. divided into 2–4 doses; in meningitis: 150 mg/kg/day i.v. divided into 3 doses

• Neonates >1 week old	25–50 mg/kg/day p.o. divided into 3–4 doses (body weight under 1,200 g: 25–50 mg/kg/day divided into 2 doses), 100 mg/kg/day i.m., i.v. divided into 3 doses; in meningitis: 200–400 mg/kg/day i.v. divided into 4 doses
In renal insufficiency (adults):	With CrCl <30 ml/min, reduction to $2/3$ of normal dose; with CrCl <20 ml/min, to $1/3$ of normal dose

In renal insufficiency (children):

CrCl	Dose (% of normal dose)
40	100
20	50 (divided into 3 doses)
10	25 (divided into 3 doses)
Anuria	15 (1–2 doses) or 30 after HD

Adverse effects:
Gastrointestinal symptoms, diarrhoea, exanthema (on average 8%; maculopapular rash in patients with infectious mononucleosis, other viral diseases and lymphocytic leukaemia), fever, rarely increased transaminases, interstitial nephritis

Contraindications:
Penicillin allergy, infectious mononucleosis and chronic lymphocytic leukaemia (in >50% of exanthemas)

Ampicillin/Sulbactam (Sultamicillin)
Alfasid® (TR), Begalin® (GR), Dicapen® (GB), Unacid® (DE, PT), Unacim® (FR), Unasyn® (AT, CZ, DE, ES, GB, IT, PL)

Spectrum:
Gram-positive, Gram-negative bacteria, particularly *H. influenzae* and Acinetobacter, β-lactamase-forming pathogens, anaerobes

Dosage:

- Adults   0.75–3 g i.v., i.m. q6–8h
- Children   150 mg/kg/day i.v. divided into 3–4
  >2 weeks old   doses
- Premature babies 75 mg/kg/day i.v. divided into 2 doses
  and neonates in
  1st week of life

In renal insufficiency (adults):	CrCl	Max. dose (g)	DI (h)
	120	3	6–8
	45	3	6–8
	18	3	12
	8	3	24
	2	3	48

In renal insufficiency (children):	CrCl	Dose (% of normal dose)
	40	75 (divided into 3 doses)
	20	50 (divided into 2 doses)
	10	30 (divided into 2 doses)
	Anuria	10 (single dose)

Adverse effects:
Gastrointestinal symptoms, diarrhoea, exanthema (on average 8%, especially in patients with infectious mononucleosis and other viral diseases, lymphocytic leukaemia), fever, rarely increased transaminases, interstitial nephritis

Contraindications:
Penicillin allergy, infectious mononucleosis and chronic lymphocytic leukaemia (exanthema formation); use during pregnancy and lactation only after painstaking benefit–risk analysis

Remarks:
The oral agent is commercially available as Sultamicillin (Unacid PD®)

- Adults   375–750 mg p.o. q12h
- Children   50 mg/kg/day divided into two doses

Anidulafungin
Ecalta® (AT, DE, DK, ES, FI, FR, GB, IS, NO, SE)

Spectrum:
Candida species including azole- and amphotericin B-resistant species, *Aspergillus* species

Dosage:

• Adults	200 mg i.v. in one dose on day 1, 100 mg i.v. in one dose from day 2
• Children	Systemic exposure after maintenance dose of 1.5 mg/kg daily comparable with adult dose of 100 mg daily
In renal insufficiency or hepatic insufficiency (all grades):	No dose adjustment necessary; anidulafungin can be given independent of the time of dialysis

Adverse effects:
Allergic reactions, raised liver values, diarrhoea, headache, nausea

Contraindications:
Hypersensitivity; not advised in pregnancy; during lactation only after benefit–risk analysis; insufficient data on efficacy and tolerability in children

Remarks:
Very slight interaction potential

Azithromycin
Azitromax® (NO, SE), Azitrox® (CZ, PL), Zithromax® (AT, BE, DE, ES, FI, FR, GB, GR, NL, PT), Zitromax® (IT, TR, DK)

Spectrum:
Staphylococci, streptococci, pneumococci, *Corynebacterium diphtheriae*, mycoplasmas, *Bordetella pertussis*, legionellae, chlamydiae, *H. influenzae, Moraxella catarrhalis*, gonococci, *Borrelia burgdorferi, Campylobacter*, relatively frequently resistant staphylococci

Dosage:

• Adults	500 mg p.o. q24h for 3 days. The total dose of 1.5 g (children: 30 mg/kg) can also be given over 5 days In pneumonia acquired outside the hospital and uncomplicated ascending adnexitis: 500 mg i.v. q24h over 2 days, then 500 mg p.o. q24h over 5–8 days
• Children	10 mg/kg p.o. q24h for 3 days
In renal insufficiency:	No dose reduction necessary

Adverse effects:
Gastrointestinal effects (3–6%), arrhythmias, rarely raised liver function parameters, in high doses hearing impairment, dizziness, ringing in the ears

Contraindications:
Severely impaired liver function, hypersensitivity to macrolides

Remarks:
For urogenital chlamydial or gonococcal infection, 1 g azithromycin (single dose)

Aztreonam
Azactam® (AT, BE, CZ, DE, DK, ES, FI, FR, GB, GR, IT, NL, NO, PL, PT, SE, TR), Primbactam® (IT)

Spectrum:
Very good in vitro activity against Gram-negative bacteria, incl. *Ps. aeruginosa*; ineffective against Gram-positive bacteria and anaerobes

Dosage:

• Adults	0.5–2 g i.v. q8–12h; i.m. only up to 1 g q8h
• Children >2 years	150–200 mg/kg/day i.v. in 3–4 doses
• Children >1 week old	90–120 mg/kg/day i.v. in 3–4 doses
In renal insufficiency (adults):	With CrCl <30 ml/min, reduction to ½ of normal dose; with CrCl <10 ml/min, reduction to ¼ of normal dose

In renal insufficiency (children):

CrCl	Dose (% of normal dose)
40	75 (divided into 3 doses)
20	50 (divided into 2 doses)
10	25 (divided into 2 doses)
Anuria	15 (single dose)

Adverse effects:
Allergic reaction, gastrointestinal symptoms, renal function impairment, increased transaminases, rarely blood count changes, peripheral and central nervous symptoms

Contraindications:
Accurate diagnosis imperative during pregnancy and lactation

Remarks:
In severe liver disease, reduce dose to 20–25% of normal. Rarely cross-allergy with penicillins or cephalosporins. Synergy with gentamicin against *Ps. aeruginosa* and *K. pneumoniae*

Caspofungin
Cancidas® (AT, BE, CZ, DE, DK, ES, FI, FR, GB, IT, NL, NO, PL, SE)

Spectrum:
Candida species including azole- and amphotericin B-resistant species, *Aspergillus* species. In vitro testing and limits have not yet been established; the published in vitro data do not permit evaluation of the sensitivity for other fungal pathogens

Dosage:

- Adults   70 mg i.v.q24h on day 1,
                    <80 kg: 50 mg q24h from day 2,
                    >80 kg: 70 mg q24h from day 2

- Children   70 mg/m^2 body surface i.v. q24h on day 1;
  >1 year   50 mg/m^2 body surface i.v. q24h on day 2.
                    If well tolerated increase the dosage to 70
                    mg/m^2 body surface q24h on day 3

In renal   No dose adjustment necessary
insufficiency:

Adverse effects:
Fever, phlebitis, headache, diarrhoea, nausea, vomiting, chills, elevated transaminases, anaemia, tachycardia

Contraindications:
During pregnancy and lactation, only after benefit–risk analysis; no data exist on suitability and efficacy in children

Remarks:
First representative of the echinocandins, a new class of antimycotics with broad spectrum of activity and good tolerability. Reduced dose to 35 mg i.v. in patients with moderate hepatic insufficiency. Calculation of body surface according to Mosteller equation (m^2):

$$\sqrt{height (cm) \times weight (kg)} \times 1/3600$$

Cefaclor
Alfatil® (FR), Altaclor® (IT), Bacticlor® (GB), Ceclor® (AT, BE, CZ, ES, GR, HR, HU, NL, PL, PT, TR), Panoral® (DE)

Spectrum:
Gram-positive (not enterococci) and Gram-negative bacteria (particularly *E. coli*, *Proteus mirabilis*, *Klebsiella*, *Haemophilus*), not for *Pseudomonas*, *Serratia*, indole-positive *Proteus*, *Enterobacter*, *Acinetobacter*

Dosage:

• Adults	0.5 g p.o. q8h (streptococci, pneumococci); 1 g p.o. q8h (Gram-neg. pathogens and *S. aureus*)
• Children >1 year old	20–40 mg/kg/day p.o. divided into 3 doses
In renal insufficiency (adults and children):	Cefaclor can be given without dose adjustment in restricted renal function. In haemodialysis patients the normal dose of cefaclor must not be altered

Adverse effects:
Nausea, vomiting, diarrhoea, allergies. Rarely: leukopenia, elevated transaminases, interstitial nephritis

Contraindications:
Cephalosporin allergy

Remarks:
Do not use in patients with known anaphylactic reaction to penicillins

---

Cefadroxil
Baxan® (GB), Biodroxil® (AT, CZ, GR, PL, PT), Cefadril® (IT), Cefamox® (SE), Cefroxil® (ES), Duracef® (BE, FI, HR, HU), Grüncef® (DE), Moxacef® (BE, GR, NL), Oracéfal® (FR)

Spectrum:
Gram-positive (not enterococci) and Gram-negative bacteria (particularly *E. coli*, *Proteus mirabilis*, *Klebsiella*), not for *Pseudomonas*, *Serratia*, indole-positive *Proteus*, *Enterobacter*, *Acinetobacter*

Dosage:

- Adults
- Children
  >1 year old
- Neonates
  >1 month old

1 g p.o. q24h

50–100 mg/kg/day p.o. divided into 2 doses; in tonsillitis ½ dose q24h

50 mg/kg/day p.o. divided into 2 doses

In renal insufficiency (adults):	CrCl	Max. dose (g)	DI (h)
	>50	1.0	12
	25–50	0.5	12
	10–25	0.5	24
	0–10	0.5	36

In renal insufficiency (children):	CrCl	Dose (% of normal dose)
	40	50 (divided into 2 doses)
	20	35 (single dose)
	10	25 (single dose)
	Anuria	15 (single dose)

Adverse effects:
Nausea, vomiting, diarrhoea, allergies. Rarely: eosinophilia, leukopenia, elevated transaminases, interstitial nephritis, headache

Contraindications:
Cephalosporin allergy

Remarks:
Do not use in patients with known anaphylactic reaction to penicillins
Resorption not affected by simultaneous intake of nutrition

Cefalexin
Cefalexina® (IT), Cefaclen® (CZ), Cefadina® (ES), Cefalin® (FR, HR), Cephalexin® (DE), Ceporex® (BE, FR), Kefalex® (FI), Keflex® (AT, DK, GB, GR, NO, PL, PT, SE), Keforal® (NL)

Spectrum:
Gram-positive (not enterococci!) and Gram-negative bacteria (particularly *E. coli*, *Proteus mirabilis*, *Klebsiella*), not for *Pseudomonas*, *Serratia*, indole-positive *Proteus*, *Enterobacter*, *Acinetobacter*

Dosage:

- Adults   0.5–1 g p.o. q6–12h
- Children   50–100 mg/kg/day p.o. divided into 2–4
  >1 year old   doses
- Neonates   40–60 mg/kg/day p.o. divided into 3 doses

In renal insufficiency (adults):	CrCl	Max. dose (g)	DI (h)
	>30	0.5	4–6
	15–30	0.5	8–12
	4–15	0.5	24

In renal	CrCl	Dose (% of normal dose)
insufficiency	40	100
(children):	20	50 (divided into 2 doses)
	10	25 (single dose)
	Anuria	20 (single dose)

Adverse effects:
Nausea, vomiting, diarrhoea, allergies. Rarely: eosinophilia, leukopenia, elevated transaminases, interstitial nephritis, headache

Contraindications:
Cephalosporin allergy

Remarks:
Do not use in patients with known anaphylactic reaction to penicillins.
Because of poor efficacy against *H. influenzae* and *Moraxella catarrhalis*, insufficient effect in otitis media and sinusitis. Resorption little affected by simultaneous intake of nutrition

---

Cefazolin
Areuzolin® (ES), Biofazolin® (PL), Biozolin® (GR), Céfacidal® (BE, FR, NL), Cefamezin® (PT, TR), Cefazil® (IT), Cephazolin fresenius® (DE), Kefzol® (AT, BE, CZ, HR, NL, TR)

Spectrum:
Gram-positive (not enterococci!) and Gram-negative bacteria (particularly *E. coli*, *Proteus mirabilis*, *Klebsiella*), not for *Pseudomonas*, *Serratia*, indole-positive *Proteus*, *Enterobacter*, *Acinetobacter*

Dosage:
- Adults   0.5–1.0 g i.m., i.v. q8–12h (Gram-pos. pathogens);
1.0 g–2.0 g i.m., i.v. q8–12h (Gram-neg. pathogens)

• Children >1 year old	50–100 mg/kg/day i.v. divided into 2–3 doses	
• Children <1 year old	25–50 mg/kg/day i.v. divided into 3–4 doses	

In renal insufficiency (adults):	CrCl	Max. dose (g)	DI (h)
	35–54	1	8
	10–34	0.5	12
	<10	0.5	18–24

In renal insufficiency (children):	CrCl	Dose (% of normal dose)
	40	75 (divided into 3 doses)
	20	50 (divided into 3 doses)
	10	30 (divided into 2 doses)
	Anuria	10 (single dose)

Adverse effects:
Nausea, vomiting, diarrhoea, allergies. Rarely: eosinophilia, leukopenia, elevated transaminases, interstitial nephritis, headache, thrombophlebitis

Contraindications:
Cephalosporin allergy

Remarks:
Do not use in patients with known anaphylactic reaction to penicillins. Do not administer intraventricularly, because of high risk of seizures

---

Cefepime
Axepim® (FR), Maxipime® (AT, BE, CZ, DE, ES, FI, GR, HR, IT, NL, PL, PT, SE, TR)

Spectrum:
Very good efficacy against Gram-positive and Gram-negative bacteria, above all *Ps. aeruginosa*, indole-positive *Proteus*, *Serratia*, *Enterobacter*, *Citrobacter*. Very good efficacy against

staphylococci, also effective against ceftazidime-resistant Gram-positive and Gram-negative bacteria

Dosage:

• Adults and adolescents >12 years	2 g i.v. q12h (q8h in serious infections)
• Infants, children >2 months	50 mg/kg i.v. q12h (q8h in serious infections)
• Infants >1 month	30 mg/kg i.v. q12h (q8h in serious infections)
In renal insufficiency (adults):	With CrCl of 30–10 ml/min, 1–2 g i.v. q24h; with CrCl under 10 ml/min, 0.5–1 g i.v. q24h. After haemodialysis 1 g i.v.

In renal insufficiency (children):	CrCl	Dose (% of normal dose)
	40	50 (1–2 doses)
	20	25 (single dose)
	10	15 (single dose)
	Anuria	15 (single dose)

Adverse effects:
Diarrhoea, thrombophlebitis, allergic reactions, fever, blood count alterations, elevated transaminases, positive Coombs test, renal function impairment, especially in combination with aminoglycosides and strong diuretics, headache, paresthesias

Contraindications:
Cephalosporin allergy and hypersensitivity to arginine

Remarks:
Do not use in patients with known anaphylactic reaction to penicillins

Cefixime
Aerocef® (AT), Bonocef® (PT), Ceftoral® (GR), Cephoral® (DE), Denvar® (ES), Oroken® (FR), Supracef® (FI), Suprax® (CZ, GB, HU, IT, TR), Tricef® (SE)

Spectrum:
Very good efficacy against streptococci, *H. influenzae* and other Gram-negative bacteria; not: *S. aureus*, *Pseudomonas*, enterococci

Dosage:

• Adults	400 mg p.o. q24h or 200 mg p.o. q12h
• Children	4 mg/kg q12h or 8 mg/kg/day p.o. q24h
In renal insufficiency (adults):	With CrCl >20 ml/min, no dose adjustment necessary; with CrCl <20 ml/min, ½ of normal dose

In renal insufficiency (children):	CrCl	Dose (% of normal dose)
	40	100
	20	50 (single dose)
	10	50 (single dose)
	Anuria	50 (single dose)

Adverse effects:
Nausea, vomiting, diarrhoea, allergies. Rarely: eosinophilia, leukopenia, elevated transaminases, nephrotoxicity, headache

Contraindications:
Cephalosporin allergy

Remarks:
Do not use in patients with known anaphylactic reaction to penicillins. Only 40–50% resorption

Cefotaxime
Biotaksym® (PL), Claforan® (AT, BE, CZ, DE, DK, ES, GB, IT, FI, FR, GR, HU, NL, NO, SE, TR)

Spectrum:
Very good efficacy against streptococci, *H. influenzae* and other Gram-negative bacteria; not staphylococci, *Pseudomonas*, enterococci

Dosage:

• Adults	1–4 g i.v. q12h (q8h in severe infections)
• Children >1 year old	50–100 mg/kg/day i.v. divided into 2–3 doses
Neonates	50–100 mg/kg/day i.v. divided into 2 doses (also for body weight under 1,200 g)
In renal insufficiency (adults):	With CrCl 5–10 ml/min, ½ of normal dose; with CrCl <5 ml/min, max. 1 g in 2 doses

In renal insufficiency (children):

CrCl	Dose (% of normal dose)
40	100
20	60 (divided into 2 doses)
10	50 (divided into 2 doses)
Anuria	50 (divided into 2 doses)

Adverse effects:
Gastrointestinal disturbances, thrombophlebitis, exanthema, fever, eosinophilia, elevated transaminases, anaphylaxis, positive Coombs test, nephrotoxicity, particularly in combination with aminoglycosides

Contraindications:
Cephalosporin allergy

Remarks:
Do not use in patients with known anaphylactic reaction to penicillins. Metabolite less effective. In the case of severe liver disease, other antibiotics should be used. A quantity of 1 g cefotaxime corresponds to 2.1 mmol sodium

---

Cefotiam
Halospor® (AT), Spizef® (AT, DE), Taketiam® (FR)

Spectrum:
For Gram-positive pathogens, more effective than cefoxitin and approximately equivalent to cefuroxime; more active than cefuroxime, cefoxitin and cefazolin against *E. coli*, *Klebsiella*, *Shigella*, *Proteus mirabilis*, *Salmonella* and *Enterobacter*; very effective against β-lactamase-forming strains of *H. influenzae*, *N. gonorrhoeae* and *S. aureus*

Dosage:

- Adults and children >12 years

  1–2 g i.v., i.m. q12h (q8h) in uncomplicated infections with sensitive pathogens
  3–4 g i.v., i.m. q12h (q8h) in moderate to severe infections and with moderately sensitive pathogens

- Children >3 months

  50–100 mg/kg/day i.v. divided into 2 doses

- Neonates 0–3 days

  40–60 mg/kg/day i.v. divided into 2–3 doses

- Neonates >4 days

  60–80 mg/kg/day i.v. divided into 3–4 doses

In renal insufficiency (adults):

CrCl	Max. dose (g)	DI (h)
120	2	12
45	2	12
18	1.5	12
8	1	12
2	1	24
0.5	0.5–1	24

In renal insufficiency (children):	CrCl	Dose (% of normal dose)
	40	100 (divided into 2 doses)
	20	75 (divided into 2 doses)
	10	50 (divided into 2 doses)
	Anuria	20 (single dose)

Adverse effects:
Gastrointestinal disturbances, thrombophlebitis, exanthema, fever, eosinophilia, elevated transaminases, leukopenia, thrombopenia, anaphylaxis, positive Coombs test, nephrotoxicity, particularly in combination with aminoglycosides

Contraindications:
Cephalosporin allergy

Remarks:
Do not use in patients with known anaphylactic reaction to penicillins

---

Cefpodoxime proxetil
Biocef® (AT), Orelox® (CZ, DE, DK, ES, FR, GB, GR, IT, NL, SE)

Spectrum:
Very good in vitro activity against Gram-positive and Gram-negative pathogens, also *H. influenzae;* not: *Ps. aeruginosa*, enterococci, staphylococci

Dosage:

• Adults	100–200 mg p.o. q12h		
• Children	5–12 mg/kg/day p.o. divided into 2 doses		

In renal insufficiency (adults):	CrCl	Max. dose (g)	DI (h)
	10–40	0.1–0.2	24
	<10	0.1–0.2	48

With haemodialysis: initially 100–200 mg, then 100–200 mg after every dialysis

In renal insufficiency (children):	CrCl	Dose (% of normal dose)
	40	75 (divided into 2 doses)
	20	50 (single dose)
	10	25 (single dose)
	Anuria	50 after HD

Adverse effects:
Nausea, vomiting, diarrhoea, allergies. Rarely: eosinophilia, leukopenia, elevated transaminases, headache

Contraindications:
Cephalosporin allergy

Remarks:
Do not use in patients with known anaphylactic reaction to penicillins
Resorption rate 40–50% (higher with intake of nutrition)
Not in neonates

Ceftazidime
Cefortam® (PT), Ceftazidim® (DE), Fortam® (ES), Fortum® (AT, CZ, DE, DK, FR, GB, NL, NO, PL, SE, TR), Ftazidime® (GR), Glazidim® (BE, FI, IT)

Spectrum:
Very good efficacy against Gram-negative bacteria, above all *Ps. aeruginosa*, indole-positive *Proteus* and *Serratia*; low efficacy against staphylococci in vitro

Dosage:

- Adults   1–2 g i.v. q8–12h
- Children   30–100 mg/kg/day i.v. divided into 2–3 doses
- Neonates   25–60 mg/kg/day i.v. divided into 2 doses (also for body weight under 1,200 g)

In renal insufficiency (adults):	CrCl	Max. dose (g)	DI (h)
	50–31	1	12
	30–16	1	24
	15–6	0.5	24
	≤5	0.5	48

In renal insufficiency (children):	CrCl	Dose (% of normal dose)
	40	50 (divided into 2 doses)
	20	25 (single dose)
	10	15 (single dose)
	Anuria	10 (single dose) or 30 after HD

Adverse effects:
Gastrointestinal disturbances, thrombophlebitis, exanthema, fever, eosinophilia, elevated transaminases, leukopenia, thrombopenia, anaphylaxis, positive Coombs test, nephrotoxicity, particularly in combination with aminoglycosides and strong diuretics

Contraindications:
Cephalosporin allergy

Remarks:
Do not use in patients with known anaphylactic reaction to penicillins. Metabolically stable, very β-lactamase stable

---

Ceftibuten
Biocef® (ES), Caedax® (AT, GR, PT), Cedax® (ES, HR, HU, IT, NL, PL, SE), Keimax® (DE)

Spectrum:
Gram-positive (not staphylococci and enterococci) and Gram-negative pathogens (particularly *H. influenzae*, *E. coli*, *Proteus*, *Klebsiella*, *M. catarrhalis*); not *Ps. aeruginosa*

Dosage:

- Adults   400 mg/day p.o. in a single dose
- Children   9 mg/kg/day p.o. in a single dose
  >3 months old

In renal insufficiency (adults):	CrCl	Max. dose (g)	DI (h)
	≥50	0.4	24
	30–49	0.2	24
	5–29	0.1	24

In renal insufficiency (children):	CrCl	Dose (% of normal dose)
	40	75 (single dose)
	20	40 (single dose)
	10	20 (single dose)
	Anuria	20 (single dose)

Adverse effects:
Nausea, vomiting, diarrhoea, headache, allergies. Rarely: eosinophilia, leukopenia, elevated transaminases, nephrotoxicity

Contraindications:
Cephalosporin allergy

Remarks:
Cross-allergy with other β-lactam antibiotics (e.g. penicillin) can occur
Resorption decreased by intake of nutrition

Ceftriaxone
Axobat® (IT), Lendacin® (CZ), Rocefalin® (ES), Rocefin® (IT), Rocephalin® (DK, FI, NO, SE), Rocephin® (AT, DE, GB, GR, HR, NL, PL, PT, TR), Rocéphine® (FR, BE)

Spectrum:
Very good efficacy against Gram-negative bacteria, except *Ps. aeruginosa*; low efficacy against staphylococci in vitro

Dosage:

• Adults and children >12 years	1–2 g i.v., i.m. q24h (Meningitis: 2 g i.v. q12h)
• Patients > 65 years	1 g i.v. q24h
• Children >1 year old	20–80 mg/kg/day i.v. as single dose
• Neonates	up to 50 mg/kg/day i.v. as single dose (also for body weight under 1,200 g)
• Neonates >1 week old	20–80 mg/kg/day i.v. as single dose
In renal insufficiency (adults):	No dose reduction necessary in moderately restricted renal function. With CrCl <10 ml/min, do not exceed a daily dose of 1 to max. 2 g

In renal insufficiency (children):

CrCl	Dose (% of normal dose)
40	100
20	100
10	80 (single dose)
Anuria	50 (single dose) or 100 after HD

Adverse effects:

Gastrointestinal disturbances, thrombophlebitis, exanthema, fever, eosinophilia, elevated transaminases, leukopenia, thrombopenia, anaphylaxis, positive Coombs test, rarely creatinine increase, reversible precipitations in gallbladder and kidney, in rare cases with clinical symptoms (pain!). Ceftriaxone and calcium-containing products should not be administered within 48 hours following each other for high risk of serious cardiopulmonary adverse events.

Contraindications:

Cephalosporin allergy

Remarks:
Do not use in patients with known anaphylactic reaction to penicillins. In the case of accompanying severe kidney and liver damage the blood plasma concentration should be monitored regularly or other antibiotics should be used. High β-lactamase stability

---

Cefuroxime
Cecim® (HU), Cefurin® (IT), Curoxima® (ES), Ketocef® (HR), Zinacef® (BE, CZ, DE, DK, FI, GB, GR, NL, NO, PL, SE, TR)

Spectrum:
As for cefotiam

Dosage:

• Adults	0.75–1.5 g i.v. q8–12h (Gram-pos. pathogens); 1.5 g i.v. q6–12h (Gram-neg. pathogens)
• Children >1 year old	30–100 mg/kg/day i.v. divided into 3–4 doses
• Premature babies and neonates	30–100 mg/kg/day i.v. divided into 2 doses

In renal insufficiency (adults):	CrCl	Max. dose (g)	DI (h)
	120	1.5	8
	45	1.5	8
	18	0.75	12
	8	0.75	12
	2	0.75	12
	0.5	0.5	24

In renal insufficiency	CrCl	Dose (% of normal dose)
(children):	40	100
	20	60 (divided into 2 doses)
	10	50 (divided into 2 doses)
	Anuria	15 (single dose) or 30 after HD

Adverse effects:
Gastrointestinal disturbances, thrombophlebitis, exanthema, fever, eosinophilia, elevated transaminases, leukopenia, thrombopenia, anaphylaxis, positive Coombs test, nephrotoxicity particularly in combination with aminoglycosides

Contraindications:
Cephalosporin allergy

Remarks:
Do not use in patients with known anaphylactic reaction to penicillins
Beware! Simultaneous administration of furosemide increases the nephrotoxicity
Less effective than cefalotin and cefazolin against staphylococci

---

Cefuroxime axetil
Cefurobac® (AT), Cepazine® (FR), Elobact® (DE), Interbion® (GR), Zinnat® (AT, BE, CZ, DK, ES, FI, FR, GB, HR, HU, IT, NL, PL, SE, TR)

Spectrum:
Gram-positive (not enterococci!) and Gram-negative bacteria (particularly *E. coli, Proteus mirabilis, Klebsiella, Borrelia burgdorferi*); not for *Pseudomonas, Serratia,* indole-positive *Proteus, Enterobacter, Acinetobacter*; very good efficacy against *H. influenzae* and moraxellae

Dosage:

- Adults and children >12 years   125–500 mg p.o. q12h

- Children >3 months old   20–30 mg/kg/day p.o. divided into 2 doses

In renal insufficiency (adults):   Can be used without dose adjustment in all degrees of renal function impairment, provided the daily dose does not exceed 1 g

In renal insufficiency (children):

CrCl	Dose (% of normal dose)
40	100
20	50 (single dose)
10	33 (single dose)
Anuria	25 (single dose)

Adverse effects:
Nausea, vomiting, diarrhoea, allergies. Rarely: eosinophilia, leukopenia, elevated transaminases, headache

Contraindications:
Cephalosporin allergy

Remarks:
Do not use in patients with known anaphylactic reaction to penicillins
Resorption best after meals (50–60%)

Chloramphenicol
Chlorocid® (HU), Chloromycetin® (AT, DK, ES, FI, GB, PT, SE), Cloramfenicolo® (IT), Cloranic® (GR), Globenicol® (NL)

Spectrum:
Gram-positive and Gram-negative pathogens, rickettsiae, anaerobes

Dosage:

- Adults and children >12 years   40–80 mg/kg/day i.v. in 3–4 doses

- Children 7–12 years   50–80 mg/kg/day i.v. in 3–4 doses

- Children 2–6 years   50–100 mg/kg/day i.v. in 3–4 doses

- Infants >4 weeks   50–100 mg/kg/day i.v. in 4 doses

Premature babies and neonates   25–50 mg/kg/day i.v. in 1–2 doses

In renal insufficiency (adults and children):   No dose adjustment necessary

Adverse effects:
Gastrointestinal symptoms, leukopenia, thrombopenia, anaemia, aplastic anaemia (1:10,000–20,000), Grey syndrome, fever, exanthema, elevated transaminases, jaundice

Contraindications:
Aplastic blood diseases, severe hepatic insufficiency with jaundice, pregnancy, lactation, perinatal period

Remarks:
Now indicated only in abdominal typhus, paratyphus A and B, life-threatening infections (e.g. salmonellal sepsis or meningitis), *H. influenzae* meningitis (in ampicillin resistance), meningitis of unknown origin, brain abscess, rickettsioses; weekly determination of plasma level; monitor blood count

---

Ciprofloxacin
Aceoto® (ES), Carmicina® (PT), Cilox® (NO), Ciprinol® (CZ, HR, PL), Ciprobay® (CZ, DE, HU, PL), Ciproxin® (IT)

Spectrum:
Nearly all Gram-positive and Gram-negative pathogens, including *H. influenzae*, salmonellae, shigellae, *Yersinia, Campylobacter*, neisseriae, legionellae, *Ps. aeruginosa;* not anaer-

obes. Only moderate efficacy against enterococci, streptococci, pneumococci, staphylococci

Dosage:

- Adults   0.1–0.75 g p.o. q12h;
                         200 mg q12h to 400 mg i.v. q8h

- Children*   30 mg/kg/day i.v. divided into 3 doses
  >5 years old   (max. 1.2 g/day) 30–40 mg/kg/day p.o.
                         divided into 2 doses (max. 1.5 g/day)

* not approved for usage in children and adolescence (5–17
years), except for the treatment of cystic fibrosis. Restriction
is based on arthropathies observed in young experimental
animals.

In renal insufficiency (adults):	With CrCl 60 ml/min, max. 1 g/day p.o. or 800 mg/day i.v.; with CrCl 30 ml/min, max. 500 mg/day p.o. or 400 mg/day i.v.

In renal insufficiency (children):	CrCl	Dose (% of normal dose)
	40	100
	20	50 (single dose)
	10	50 (single dose)
	Anuria	33 (single dose)

Adverse effects:
Gastrointestinal symptoms, CNS disturbances (e.g. visual impairments, dizziness, cramps, sleeplessness, psychotic disturbances), allergies, joint pains, altered blood count and laboratory parameters, QT interval prolongation, interstitial nephritis, tendinitis

Contraindications:
Pregnancy and lactation, children and adolescents (exception:
mucoviscidosis)

Remarks:
Increased resistance, above all for *S. aureus* and *Ps. aeruginosa*. Sole indication in children and adolescents: infections of the airways in mucoviscidosis. No dose adaptation required in hepatic insufficiency. Painstaking benefit–risk analysis in patients with epilepsy and other previous CNS lesions; oral bioavailability 70–80%. Avoid concomitant drugs with potential to QT interval prolongation

Clarithromycin
Biclar® (BE), Claromycin® (GR), Klacid® (AT, CZ, DE, DK, ES, FI, HR, IT, NL, NO, PL, PT, SE, TR)

Spectrum:
Gram-positive and Gram-negative pathogens, particularly staphylococci, streptococci, *Helicobacter pylori, H. influenzae*, pneumococci, *Corynebacterium diphtheriae*, mycoplasmas, *B. pertussis*, legionellae, chlamydiae, *Campylobacter, Mycobacterium avium*; better efficacy than erythromycin in vitro

Dosage:

• Adults	250–500 mg p.o. q12h, 500 mg i.v. q12h
• Children	15 mg/kg/day p.o. divided into 2 doses
In renal insufficiency (adults):	No dose adjustment necessary in moderately restricted renal function. With CrCl <30 ml/min, the dose should be reduced by half. The total duration of therapy should not exceed 2 weeks. The total dose should not exceed 250 mg/day (single dose)

In renal insufficiency (children):

CrCl	Dose (% of normal dose)
40	100
20	50 (divided into 2 doses)
10	50 (divided into 2 doses)
Anuria	50 (divided into 2 doses)

Adverse effects:
Occasionally gastrointestinal symptoms, rarely hypersensitivity reactions, very rarely liver function impairment and cardiac rhythm disturbances with prolonged QT interval

Contraindications:
Severely restricted liver function, hypersensitivity to macrolides, simultaneous administration of cisapride, pimozide, terfenadine or astemizole

Remarks:
Mavid® is indicated only in AIDS patients with disseminated or local mycobacterial infections

---

Clindamycin
Cleocin® (TR), Dalacin® C (AT, BE, CZ, DK, FI, GB, HU, IT, NL, NO, PL, SE), Sobelin® (DE)

Spectrum:
Streptococci, pneumococci, staphylococci, *Bacteroides fragilis* (ca. 9% resistance) and other anaerobes

Dosage:

• Adults	150–450 mg p.o. q6–8h; 200–600 mg i.v. q6–8h
• Children >4 weeks	8–25 mg/kg/day p.o. divided into 3–4 doses; 15–40 mg/kg/day i.v. divided into 3–4 doses
In renal insufficiency (adults and children):	Clindamycin's half-life is not extended in restricted renal function and it can be given at the normal dosage regardless of the degree of impairment. With CrCl <10 ml/min, clindamycin may accumulate

Adverse effects:
Pseudomembranous enterocolitis, exanthema, leukopenia, elevated transaminases, diarrhoea in up to 20%, thrombophlebitis, rarely allergic reactions

Contraindications:
Hypersensitivity to lincosamides; parenterally in young infants (large amount of benzyl alcohol as conservation medium)

Remarks:
An agent of choice for anaerobic infections. Do not inject undiluted

---

Colistin
Colimicina® (IT, ES), Colimycin® (DK, NO), Colimycine® (BE, FR), Colistin® (AT, DE, GR, PL), Colomycin® (GB)

Spectrum:
Gram-negative bacteria, particularly *Ps. aeruginosa* (not: *Proteus* species and *Serratia*)

Dosage:

- Adults

  1 million IU q12h to 2 million IU i.v. q8h (80–160 mg g8h; 4–6 mg/kg day); 30,000 IU/kg/day for inhalation; 4 tablets q6h to 500,000 IU p.o. (to SDD)

- Children >1 year old

  2 tablets. p.o. q6–8h

In renal insufficiency (adults):	CrCl	Max. dose (mg/kg)	DI (h)
	50–80	2.5–3.8	24
	10–50	1.5–2.5	24–36
	<10	0.6	24

In renal insufficiency (children):	CrCl	Dose (% of normal dose)
	40	75 (divided into 2 doses)
	20	50 (divided into 2 doses)
	10	25 (single dose)
	Anuria	25 (single dose)

Adverse effects:
Nausea, vomiting, exanthemas, urticaria; neuro- or nephro-toxic reactions possible in patients with renal insufficiency

Contraindications:
Hypersensitivity to colistin; premature and newborn infants

Remarks:
Care in the case of simultaneous administration of curarimimetic substances. Simultaneous administration of colistin i.v. and for inhalation has been proven to be efficacious in patients with pneumonia.

Cotrimoxazole (TMP/SMX)
Abactrim® (ES), Bactrim® (AT, BE, CZ, DK, FI, FR, GB, IT, NO, PL, PT, SE, TR), Eusaprim® (AT, BE, DE, IT, NL, SE)

Spectrum:
Pneumococci, staphylococci, gonococci, *E. coli*, salmonellae, shigellae, klebsiellae, *Proteus, Pneumocystis jiroveci* (*carinii*); not: enterococci, streptococci, and *Pseudomonas*

Dosage:*

- Adults   160 mg TMP/800 mg SMX p.o. q12h; 80 mg TMP/400 mg SMX i.v. q12h

- Children   160 mg TMP/800 mg SMX p.o. divided
  6–12 years   into 2 doses

- Children   80 mg TMP/400 mg SMX p.o. divided
  >6 months   into 2 doses

- Infants >6 weeks 40 mg TMP/200 mg SMX p.o. divided
                    into 2 doses

*Single-strength is 80 mg TMP/400 mg SMX; double-strength is 160 mg TMP/800 mg SMX

In renal insufficiency (adults):	CrCl	Dose
	>30	Standard dose
	15–30	½ standard dose, check plasma SMX[3]
	<15	Contraindicated

[3] The total plasma concentration of SMX should be measured 12 h after intake on the 3rd day of treatment. Therapy must be discontinued if the level rises to over 150 µg/ml

In renal insufficiency (children):	CrCl	Dose (% of normal dose)
	40	100
	20	100 for 3 days, then 20 (single dose)
	10	Contraindicated
	Anuria	Contraindicated

Adverse effects:
Steven–Johnson syndrome, rarely allergy, gastrointestinal symptoms, thrombopenia, leukopenia, agranulocytosis; serious adverse effects more common in patients >60 years.

Contraindications:
Sulfonamide hypersensitivity, first month of life, acute hepatitis, some haemoglobinopathies, megaloblastic anaemia because of folic acid deficiency, blood dyscrasias, high-grade renal insufficiency, severe liver damage

Remarks:
One of the agents of choice in urinary tract infections, shigellosis, nocardiosis, long-term excreters of typhus and paratyphus, abdominal typhus, paratyphus A and B. Follow manu-

facturer's instructions for i.v. administration. New TMP/sulfonamide combinations have no appreciable advantage. *Pneumocystis jiroveci (carinii)* pneumonia: 4–5 times normal dose (20 mg/kg TMP, 100 mg/kg SMX); i.v. for the first 24 h

---

Daptomycin
Cubicin® (AT, DE, ES, FR, GB, IT, NO, PT, SE)

Spectrum:
Gram-positive pathogens incl. multiresistant bacteria; particularly staphylococci (incl. MRSA, MRSE), streptococci and enterococci (incl. VRE)

Dosage:

• Adults	Complicated skin and soft tissue infections: 4 mg/kg i.v. q24h brief infusion over 30 min Bacteraemia, infectious endocarditis: 6 mg/kg i.v. q24h brief infusion over 30 min
• Children	There are no data on use in children
In renal insufficiency:	With CrCl ≥30 ml/min, no dose adjustment is necessary; with CrCl <30 ml/min, 4 mg/kg as single dose q48h. With haemodialysis the dose is given directly after dialysis

Adverse effects:
Gastrointestinal symptoms (nausea, obstipation, diarrhoea), reactions at the injection site, headache, sleep disturbances, rash, reversible increase in liver parameters and CK, myalgia

Contraindications:
Hypersensitivity to daptomycin

Remarks:
First representative of a completely new class of antibiotics (cyclic lipopeptides), new mechanism of action. Bactericidal action. No cross-resistance to other antibiotics. Monitor CK levels at least weekly

---

Dicloxacillin
Diclocil® (DK, FI, GR, NL, NO, PT, SE)

Spectrum:
Staphylococci

Dosage:

• Adults	0.5 g p.o. q4–6h (max. 4) g/day
• Children 1–6 years	0.25 g p.o. q4–6h (max. 2) g/day
• Infants >3 months	0.125–0.25 g p.o. q6h (max. 1) g/day
• Infants	30–50 mg/kg p.o. q8h
In renal insufficiency (adults):	With CrCl<30 ml/min, dose reduction. In terminal renal insufficiency the daily dose should not exceed 1 g p.o. q8h

In renal insufficiency (children):	CrCl	Dose (% of normal dose)
	40	100 (divided into 4 doses)
	20	75 (divided into 4 doses)
	10	60 (divided into 3 doses)
	Anuria	30 (single dose)

Adverse effects:
Diarrhoea, fever, exanthema, elevated transaminases, leukopenia. Rarely: interstitial nephritis (haematuria), eosinophilia

Contraindications:
Penicillin allergy

Doripenem
Doribax® (AT, DE, ES, FI, GB, NO, SE)

Spectrum:
Very good in vitro activity against Gram-positive (non-methicillin-resistant *S. aureus* and *E. faecium*) and Gram-negative bacteria incl. *Pseudomonas* species (not: *Stenotrophomonas maltophilia*)

Dosage:

• Adults	0.5 g i.v. q8h (infusion time 1–4 hours)
• Children and adolescents (<18 years)	not recommended for use in children due to a lack of safety and efficacy data
In renal insufficiency (adults):	With CrCl of 51–79 ml/min, no dosage adjustment necessary (0.5 g q8h); with CrCl of 30 to <50 ml/min, 0.25 g q8h; with CrCl <30 ml/min, 0.25 g q12h. Use with caution in patients with severe renal impairment

Adverse effects:
Headaches, gastrointestinal symptoms, nausea, diarrhoea, allergies, pruritus, rash, anemia (frequency not known)

Contraindications:
Hypersensitivity

Remarks:
Monosubstance, additional cilastatin not necessary. Do not use in patients with known anaphylactic reaction to penicillins

Doxycycline
Actidox® (PT), Bassado® (IT), Clisemina® (ES), Dinamisin® (TR), Dotur® (PL), Doxy® (BE, FR), Doxyhexal® (DE), Vibramycin® (AT, CZ, DK, GB, GR, HR, NL, NO, SE)

Spectrum:
Gram-positive, Gram-negative pathogens, mycoplasmas, chlamydiae, borreliae, *Coxiella burnetii*, ca. 50% of *Bacteroides*; not: *Proteus* species, *Ps. aeruginosa*; relatively frequent resistance by pneumococci, streptococci, staphylococci, and Gram-negative bacteria

Dosage:

• Adults	100 mg p.o. q12h or 200 mg p.o., i.v. q24h (only in mild infections: from day 2, 100 mg p.o. q24h)
• Children >8 years old	4 mg/kg/day p.o., i.v. divided into 2 doses on day 1, from day 2 onward 2 mg/kg/day
In renal insufficiency (adults and children):	At the normal dosage of 200 mg on day 1 and then 100 mg daily, there is no accumulation of active substance even in renal insufficiency.

Adverse effects:
Gastrointestinal symptoms, exanthema, rarely anaphylaxis, hepatotoxicity, pseudotumor cerebri, nephrotoxicity; less dental discoloration and photosensitivity than with tetracycline

Contraindications:
Pregnancy; do not administer to children

Remarks:
If at all possible, i.v. administration should be limited to about 2 weeks

Enoxacin
Comprecin® (GB), Enoksetin® (TR), Enoxabion® (FI), Enoxen® (IT), Enoxor® (AT, DE, FR), Gyramid® (CZ)

Spectrum:
Almost all Gram-positive and Gram-negative pathogens, including *H. influenzae*, salmonellae, shigellae, *Yersinia, Campylobacter*, neisseriae, legionellae; not anaerobes. Only slight action against *Ps. aeruginosa*, enterococci, streptococci, pneumococci

Dosage:

• Adults	400 mg p.o. q12h (200 mg p.o. q12h in uncomplicated UTI)
In renal insufficiency (adults):	With CrCl of <30 ml/min, corresponding to serum creatinine values of 2.5–5 mg/dl, the dosage is 400 mg once daily

Adverse effects:
Gastrointestinal symptoms, occasionally headaches, dizziness, sleep disturbances, exanthema, hypogeusia, cramps, tendinitis, phototoxicity

Contraindications:
Pregnancy and lactation, epilepsy and previous CNS diseases, severe renal and hepatic insufficiency; do not administer to children and adolescents

Remarks:
Beware! Resistance is developing, particularly in *Pseudomonas* and staphylococci

Ertapenem
Invanz® (AT, CZ, DE, DK, ES, FI, FR, GB, HR, IT, NO, PL, SE)

Spectrum:
Almost all Gram-positive and Gram-negative bacteria and anaerobes; weak or no effect against *Acinetobacter, Stenotrophomonas maltophilia, Ps. aeruginosa*, MRSA, MRSE and enterococci

Dosage:

- Adults and adolescents
1 g i.v. q24h (infusion over 30 min)

- Children (3 months –12 years)
15 mg/kg i.v. q12h

In renal insufficiency:
Contraindicated with CrCl <30 ml/min (insufficient data)

Adverse effects:
Gastrointestinal disturbances, central nervous symptoms (particularly headache and dizziness), dyspnea, exanthema, pruritus, elevated transaminases, thrombocytosis; thrombophlebitis

Contraindications:
Hypersensitivity to carbapenems and other ß-lactam antibiotics

Remarks:
Better in vitro activity against *Enterobacteriaceae* than imipenem and meropenem, but practically no effect on *Ps. aeruginosa*

Erythromycin
Abboticin® (DK, FI, NO, SE), Bronsema® (ES), Eritrocina® (IT), Erythrocin® (AT, CZ, DE, GB, GR, TR), Érythrocine® (BE, FR, NL)

Spectrum:
Gram-positive pathogens, especially staphylococci, streptococci, pneumococci, *Corynebacterium diphtheria*, mycoplasmas, *B. pertussis*, legionellae, chlamydiae, *Campylobacter*, relatively frequently resistant staphylococci and *H. influenzae*

Dosage:

• Adults	250–500 mg p.o., i.v. q6–8h (max. 4 g/day)
• Children >1 year old	20–50 mg/kg/day p.o. or 15–20 mg/kg/day i.v. divided into 2–4 doses
In renal insufficiency (adults):	With moderately restricted renal function no dose reduction is necessary. In anuria the dosing interval should be increased 2- to 3-fold. The total duration of therapy should not exceed 2–3 weeks

In renal insufficiency (children):	CrCl	Dose (% of normal dose)
	40	100
	20	100
	10	60 (divided into 3 doses)
	Anuria	60 (divided into 3 doses)

Adverse effects:
Gastrointestinal symptoms, very rarely allergies, liver damage, hearing impairment, ventricular arrhythmia with prolonged QT interval; especially for erythromycin estolate, reduce dose in pregnancy and pre-existing liver disease

Contraindications:
Hypersensitivity to macrolides, treatment with terfenadine, cisapride, pimozide or carbamazepine

Ethambutol

Clobutol® (PT), EMB-Fatol® (AT, DE), Embutol® (TR), Etapi-
am® (IT), Myambutol® (AT, BE, DE, DK, ES, GB, GR, FR, NL),
Oributol® (FI), Sural® (CZ, HU)

Spectrum:

M. tuberculosis, M. kansasii, M. avium-intracellulare

Dosage:

- Adults and chil-   20–25 mg/kg/day p.o. in a single dose
  dren >10 years

- Children   25 mg/kg/day p.o. in a single dose
  >5 years

- Children   30 mg/kg/day p.o. in a single dose
  0–5 years

In renal   CrCl 30–80 ml/min: 25 mg/kg/day;
insufficiency   CrCl <30–10 ml/min: 25 mg/kg three
(adults):   times weekly;
     CrCl <10 ml/min: 25 mg/kg three times
     weekly

In renal insufficiency (children)	CrCl	Dose (% of normal dose)
	40	60 (single dose)
	20	30 (single dose)
	10	Measure concentration[4]
	Anuria	Measure concentration[4]

[4]Peak concentration 2–5 µg/ml

Adverse effects:

Optic neuritis, central scotoma, peripheral neuropathy, headache, anaphylactoid reaction

Contraindications:

Previous optic nerve damage

Remarks:

Monthly ophthalmologic examination, especially red–green differentiation and visual field restriction; ethambutol is not recommended in children under 10 years of age because vision tests are not reliable. Intermittent administration of 45–50 mg/kg twice weekly is also possible. In combination with rifampin, long-term administration of a dose of 15 mg/kg/day can be considered after an initial full dose for the first 2 months

---

Flucloxacillin

Flix® (TR), Floxapen® (AT, BE, GB, GR, NL, NO, PT), Flucinal® (IT), Heracillin® (DK, SE), Pantaflux® (IT), Staphylex® (DE, FI)

Spectrum:

Staphylococci, streptococci, *Corynebacterium diphtheria, N. meningitidis, Bacillus* species

Dosage:

• Adults	0.5–1 g p.o., i.m., i.v. q6–8h (max. 12 g/day); p.o. administration ca. 1 h before meals
• Children 10–14 years	1.5–2 g/day p.o., i.v., i.m. in 3–4 doses
• Children 6–10 years	0.75–1.5 g/day p.o., i.v., i.m. in 3–4 doses
• Premature babies, neonates, young children	40–50 (max. 100) mg/kg/day p.o., i.v., i.m. in 3 doses
In renal insufficiency (adults):	Flucloxacillin is excreted to a large extent by the kidney. The dose or the dose interval may need modification in patients with renal failure: If CrCl drops below 10 ml/min, then the recommended dosage is 1 g every 8–12 hours. In anuric pa-

tients, the maximun dosage is 1 g every 12 hours. Flucloxacillin is not significantly removed by haemodialysis or peritoneal dialysis, i.e. dialysis does not need to be accompanied by an additional dose.

In renal insufficiency (children):

CrCl	Dose (% of normal dose)
40	100
20	75 (divided into 3 doses)
10	50 (divided into 3 doses)
Anuria	25 (single dose)

Adverse effects:
Diarrhoea, fever, exanthema, Hb reduction, leukopenia, elevated transaminases; rarely interstitial nephritis (haematuria), eosinophilia, cholestatic hepatitis (risk 1:15,000)

Contraindications:
Penicillin allergy

Remarks:
Penicillinase-resistant penicillin of choice, together with dicloxacillin. Single i.m. dose should not exceed 33 mg/kg in children or in adults a total dose of 2 g

---

Fluconazole
Diflucan® (AT, BE, CZ, DE, DK, ES, GB, IT, FI, HR, HU, NL, NO, PL, PT, SE), Tierlite® (GR), Triflucan® (FR, TR)

Spectrum:
Cryptococcus neoformans, Candida species (not *C. krusei*), *Microsporum canis*; no action against *Aspergillus* species

Dosage:

• Adults	Initial dose of 400 (max. 800; in severe infection, neutropenia, max. 1600) mg p.o., i.v. q24h, then 200–400 mg p.o., i.v. q24h (for *C. glabrata* 1× 800 mg [resistance testing!]) or as brief infusion in systemic mycoses. In severe parenchymatous infections (e.g. pneumonia) 800 mg/day i.v. for the first 3 days. Mucosal, oropharyngeal and esophageal candidiasis: 200 mg i.v. loading dose then 100 mg i.v. daily. Vaginal candidiasis: single dose of 150 mg p.o.
• Children	3–6 mg/kg/day p.o. or as brief infusion; in life-threatening infection up to 12 mg/kg/day i.v. Dosing interval (according to age): <2 weeks 72 h; 2–4 weeks 48 h; >4 weeks daily administration

In renal insufficiency (adults):

CrCl	Max. dose (g)
>50	200–400
11–50	100–200
Dialysis	200–400

In renal insufficiency (children):

CrCl	Dose (% of normal dose)
40	50 (single dose)
20	80 q48h
10	100 q72h
Anuria	100 after HD

Adverse effects:

Gastrointestinal symptoms, exanthema, CNS symptoms (dizziness, cramps etc.); rarely liver function impairment, leukocytopenia, thrombocytopenia

Contraindications:
Pregnancy and lactation, severely impaired liver function, treatment with terfenadine and cisapride

Remarks:
In children under 16, fluconazole should be used only when the responsible physician deems necessary. Selection of resistant *Candida* species preferentially in AIDS patients undergoing long-term continuous therapy. Good resorption with oral intake (independent of gastric juice pH). Very good penetration of cerebrospinal fluid, thus well suited for suppression therapy of cryptococcosis in AIDS patients (for primary treatment of cryptococcal meningitis, amphotericin B in combination with flucytosine is better but is associated with multiple drug interactions)

Flucytosine
Ancotil® (AT, CZ, DE, DK, ES, FI, FR, GB, IT, NL, NO, PL, PT, SE)

Spectrum:
Good to very good efficacy against most *Candida* species, *Cryptococcus neoformans*, good effect against some *Aspergillus* species (particularly *A. fumigatus*) and bacteria causing chromoblastomycosis; not effective, for example, against *Histoplasma* and *Blastomyces*

Dosage:
- Adults and children   150–200 (max. 300) mg/kg/day i.v. in 4 doses
- Premature babies and neonates   60–80 mg/kg/day i.v. divided into 2 doses

In renal insufficiency (adults):	CrCl	Max. dose (mg/kg)	DI (h)
	>40	(25–)50	6
	20–40	(25–)50	12
	10–20	(25–)50	24
	<10	50	>24

In anuria the second dose should be a repeat of the initial dose of 50 mg/kg and should be given only after the next dialysis. The mean serum concentration should be 25–40 µg/ml

In renal insufficiency (children):	CrCl	Dose (% of normal dose)
	40	50 (divided into 2 doses)
	20	25 (single dose)
	10	20 (single dose)
	Anuria	100 after HD

Adverse effects:
Reversible blood count changes (leukopenia, thrombopenia, anaemia), irreversible bone marrow damage (in combination with immunosuppressants), temporary increase in transaminases, rarely gastrointestinal symptoms, CNS symptoms (dizziness, hallucinations etc.), photosensitivity

Contraindications:
Pregnancy; do not prescribe to neonates

Remarks:
Primary resistance is very rare (<5%) in *Candida* species, with the exception of *C. krusei*. The combination of flucytosine and amphotericin B (see p. 67 ► for dosage) is synergistic and reduces development of resistance. Do not use flucytosine prophylactically (development of resistance!). Exercise caution in the presence of renal insufficiency, liver damage and existing bone marrow depression

Fosfomycin
Fosfocin® (DK, IT) , Infectofos® (DE)

Spectrum:
Staphylococci, streptococci, gonococci, *E. faecalis, H. influenzae, E. coli, Proteus mirabilis*, salmonellae, shigellae; partially *Ps. aeruginosa* and *Serratia marcescens*

Dosage:

- Adults and
  adolescents

  6–16 g* i.v. divided into 2–3 doses
  *different maximal dosages recommended in different European countries, e.g. 4 g (FR, ES) i.v. q6h; 5 g (DE) i.v. q6h; 8 g (AT) i.v. q8h

- Children 1–12 years

  100–200 (max. 300) mg/kg/day i.v. in 3 doses

- Infants

  200–250 mg/kg/day i.v. in 3 doses

- Premature babies
  and neonates

  100 mg/kg/day i.v. in 2 doses

In renal insufficiency (adults): Intended normal dose 5 g i.v. q8h or 8 g i.v. q12 h

CrCl	Max. dose (g)	DI (h)
45	3	6
18	3	8
8	3	12
2	1.5	12
0.5	1.5	24

Intended normal dose 3 g i.v. q8h

CrCl	Max. dose (g)	DI (h)
45	3	12
18	1.5	8
8	1.5	12
2	1.5	24
0.5	1.0	24

Intended normal dose 2 g i.v. q8h	CrCl	Max. dose (g)	DI (h)
	45	2	12
	18	1	8
	8	1	12
	2	1	24
	0.5	1	36
In renal insufficiency (children):	CrCl	Dose (% of normal dose)	
	40	50 (divided into 3 doses)	
	20	30 (divided into 2 doses)	
	10	20 (divided into 2 doses)	
	Anuria	10 (single dose)	

Adverse effects:

Gastrointestinal symptoms, transient increase in liver enzymes, exanthema, phlebitis, dyspnea, headache, disturbances of taste

Contraindications:

Hypersensitivity to fosfomycin or succinic acid

Remarks:

Mechanism of action unrelated to any other antibiotic. Because of potential development of resistance during treatment, fosfomycin should be used only in combination. Monitor serum electrolytes because of the relatively high sodium loading (1 g fosfomycin corresponds to 14.5 mmol sodium). The oral formulation of fosfomycin (fosfomycin trometamol; Monuril®) is licensed solely for the treatment of uncomplicated cystitis; the tissue concentration achieved is not sufficient to combat systemic infections

Gentamicin
Cidomycin® (GB), Garamycin® (CZ, DK, FI, GR, HR, NL, NO, PL, SE, TR), Gentamicina® (IT), Refobacin® (DE)

Spectrum:
Gram-positive bacteria (staphylococci; not: pneumococci, streptococci, enterococci), Gram-negative bacteria

Dosage:

• Adults	3–6 mg/kg/day i.m., i.v. divided into 1–3 doses (30–60 min brief infusion)
• Children >1 month old	4.5–7.5 mg/kg/day i.m., i.v. divided into 3 doses
• Neonates	4–7 mg/kg/day i.m., i.v. in 1(–2) dose(s) (also for body weight under 1,200 g)

In renal insufficiency (adults):

CrCl	Max. dose (g)	DI (h)
120	0.12	8
45	0.12	12
18	0.04	12
8	0.04	24
2	0.02	24[6]
0.5	0.02	24[6, 7]

[6] In life-threatening cases, initial dose of 100 mg

[7] Two to three haemodialyses per week are considered necessary in such cases. One normal dose initially

In renal insufficiency (children):

CrCl	Dose (% of normal dose)
40	60 (divided into 2 doses)
20	20 (divided into 2 doses); LD 2–3 mg/kg
10	10 (single dose); LD 2 mg/kg 5 (single dose) or 15 after HD;
Anuria	LD 1–2 mg/kg

Adverse effects:
Ototoxicity and nephrotoxicity, particularly with peak concentration >10 µg/ml or trough concentration >2 µg/ml, with previous aminoglycoside therapy, and with simultaneous administration of furosemide or ethacrynic acid. Neuromuscular blockade, exanthema

Contraindications:
Parenteral administration in first 3 months of pregnancy; from the 4th month of gestation only in life-threatening circumstances

Remarks:
Do not mix aminoglycoside solutions with penicillins or cephalosporins (inactivation of the aminoglycosides)

Imipenem/Cilastatin
Primaxin® (GB, GR), Tienam® (BE, CZ, DK, ES, FR, FI, HR, IT, NL, NO, PL, PT, SE, TR), Zienam® (DE, AT)

Spectrum:
Very good in vitro activity against Gram-positive (not: methicillin-resistant *S. aureus* and *E. faecium*) and Gram-negative bacteria (moderate effect on *Pseudomonas* species), including anaerobes; not: *Stenotrophomonas maltophilia*

Dosage:

- Adults   0.5–1.0 g i.v. q6–8h (max. dose: 50 mg/kg or 4 g)
- Children >3 months old   60 mg/kg/day i.v. divided into 3(–4) doses (max. 2 g/day)
- Infants   50 mg/kg/day i.v. in 2–3 doses

In renal insufficiency (adults):	CrCl	Single dose (g)	DI (h)
	>70	0.5–1	6–8
	41–70	0.25–0.75	6–8
	21–40	0.25–0.5	6–8
	6–20	0.25–0.5	12
	<6	As for CrCl 6–20, if HD possible within 48 h	

In renal insufficiency (children):	CrCl	Dose (% of normal dose)
	40	75 (divided into 3 doses)
	20	50 (divided into 2 doses)
	10	25 (divided into 2 doses)
	Anuria	15 (single dose)

Adverse effects:

Exanthema, blood count changes, thrombocytosis, eosinophilia, leukopenia, elevated transaminases and alkaline phosphatase, gastrointestinal symptoms, dizziness, seizures (!), prolongation of prothrombin time, positive Coombs test

Contraindications:

Imipenem/cilastatin allergy; caution in the case of allergy to other β-lactam antibiotics

Remarks:

In severe infection, combined with another aminoglycoside. In vitro antagonism in combination with cephalosporins or broad-spectrum penicillins. For infants <3 months not approved, in case of nonresponse to other antibiotics try with 40 mg/kg/day i.v. divided into 2 doses

Isoniazid (INH)
Eutizon® (HR), Isoniazid® (HU), Isozid® (DE), Nicozid® (IT), Nidrazid® (CZ), Rimifon® (BE, FR, GB)

Spectrum:
M. tuberculosis, M. kansasii

Dosage:

• Adults	5 mg/kg/day, max. 300 mg/day in a single dose p.o. or i.v.
• Children	
• 0–5 years	10–9 mg/kg
• 6–9 years	8–7 mg/kg
• 10–14 years	7–6 mg/kg
• 15–18 years	6–5 mg/kg
	max. 300 mg/day
In renal insufficiency (adults and children):	INH is eliminated from serum independently of renal function, i.e. the biological half-life is not prolonged even in anuric patients. Even with restricted renal function a daily dose of 5 mg/kg body weight is given

Adverse effects:
Peripheral neuropathy, rarely cramps, optic neuritis, encephalopathy, psychoses, often hepatitis (frequency increases with age, average 1–2%), fever, allergic skin signs, leukopenia

Contraindications:
Acute hepatitis, psychoses, epilepsy, alcohol dependency, impaired coagulation, peripheral neuritis

Remarks:
Monitoring of liver function (transaminases) – increase seen in 20–30% of patients. Discontinue INH if transaminases >100–150 U/l

Established drug combinations for the treatment of tuberculosis are

Rifampin + isoniazid: Rifinah® (FR, IT)
Rifampin + isoniazid + pyrazinamide: Rifater® (FR, IT, ES)

Itraconazole
Canadiol® (ES), Funit® (TR), Itrac® (HR), Orungal® (HU, PL), Sempera® (DE), Sporanox® (AT, BE, CZ, DK, FI, FR, GB, GR, IT, NO, PT, SE)

Spectrum:
Broad spectrum of action against many species of fungi, very good efficacy against *Aspergillus* species

Dosage:

• Adults	200 mg p.o. q12–24h with a meal; in severe infection, LD of 200 mg p.o. q8h for 4 days, then 200 mg p.o. q12h; 200 mg i.v. q12h for 2 days, then 200 mg i.v. q24h
In renal insufficiency:	No dose reduction is necessary in various degrees of renal insufficiency. Even in dialysis patients the dosage need not be altered

Adverse effects:
Nausea, vomiting, pains, dizziness, exanthema, allergies, elevated transaminases, hypokalaemia. At higher dose (600 mg/day), hypertension, severe hypokalaemia, adrenocortical insufficiency

Contraindications:
Pregnancy and lactation; do not prescribe to children and adolescents

Remarks:

Well-tolerated azole derivative with broad antimycotic spectrum. Poor penetration of cerebrospinal fluid. Itraconazole prolongs the excretion of cyclosporine, digoxin, phenytoin and warfarin, but accelerates the metabolisation of INH, rifampin, phenobarbital, carbamazepine and phenytoin

---

Levofloxacin
Tavanic® (AT, BE, CZ, DE, ES, FI, FR, GB, GR, HR, IT, NL, PL, PT, SE, TR)

Spectrum:

Almost all Gram-positive and Gram-negative pathogens, including pneumococci, streptococci, *E. faecalis*, staphylococci, chlamydiae, *Mycoplasma pneumoniae*, legionellae, *H. influenzae, Ps. aeruginosa*; only moderately effective against anaerobes

Dosage:

• Adults	250–500 mg p.o., i.v. q12–24h
In renal insufficiency (adults):	CrCl 50–20 ml/min: normal dose on day 1, then half-normal single daily dose; CrCl <20 ml/min: normal dose on day 1, then ¼ initial dose as maintenance dose

Adverse effects:

Gastrointestinal symptoms, headaches, stupor, dizziness, somnolence, photosensitivity, tendinitis, elevated transaminases

Contraindications:

Pregnancy and lactation, epilepsy, tendon symptoms after previous use of fluoroquinolones, hypersensitivity to levofloxacin or another quinolones; do not prescribe to children or adolescents

Remarks:

No clinically relevant interaction with theophylline; caution when taken together with medications that lower the cramp threshold

Linezolid
Zyvox® (GB), Zyvoxid® (AT, BE, CZ, DE, DK, ES, FI, FR, IT, NL, NO, PL, PT, SE)

Spectrum:
Staphylococci (incl. MRSA, MRSE and GISA), streptococci (incl. penicillin-resistant pneumococci), enterococci (incl. VRE) and other Gram-positive pathogens

Dosage:

• Adults	600 mg p.o., i.v. q12h
In renal insufficiency:	No dose adjustment necessary in renal insufficiency

Adverse effects:
Mainly gastrointestinal symptoms (nausea, diarrhoea) and slight to moderate headaches, candidiasis, fungal infections, dysgeusia (metallic taste); neutropenia, anaemia, thrombocytopenia; peripheral and/or optic neuropathy, lactic acidosis

Contraindications:
Hypersensitivity to linezolid or any of its ingredients, intake of MAO inhibitors A or B currently or within previous 2 weeks; uncontrolled hypertension, pheochromocytoma, carcinoid, thyrotoxicosis, bipolar depression, schizoaffective disturbance, acute confusional states; current intake of serotonin reuptake inhibitors, tricyclic antidepressants, sympathicomimetics

Remarks:
Novel mechanism of action, complete bioavailability following oral intake, weekly blood counts especially in predisposed patients to check for anaemia and thrombocytopenia. No cross resistance to other antibiotics, little experience so far of long-term therapy (>4 weeks)

Loracarbef
Lorabid® (AT, GR, NL, SE, TR), Lorafem® (DE)

Spectrum:
Gram-positive (not enterococci) and Gram-negative bacteria (particularly *E. coli, Proteus mirabilis, Klebsiella, Moraxella catarrhalis, H. influenzae*), not: *Pseudomonas, Serratis,* indole-positive *Proteus, Enterobacter, Acinetobacter*

Dosage:

• Adults and children >12 years	200–400 mg p.o. q12h 200 mg p.o. q24h (in uncomplicated UTI in females)
• Children >6 months	15–30 mg/kg/day p.o. divided into 2 doses (maximum dose 800 mg/day)
In renal insufficiency (adults):	With CrCl of 49–10 ml/min, 200–400 mg once daily; with CrCl <10 ml/min, 200–400 mg every 3rd day

In renal insufficiency (children):	CrCl	Dose (% of normal dose)
	40	50 (single dose)
	20	50 (single dose)
	10	15 (single dose)
	Anuria	15 (single dose)

Adverse effects:
Nausea, vomiting, diarrhoea, allergies. Rarely: eosinophilia, leukopenia, elevated transaminases, nephrotoxicity, headaches

Contraindications:
Cephalosporin allergy

Remarks:
Do not use in patients with known anaphylactic reaction to penicillins. No experience to date during pregnancy and lactation: treatment only after painstaking benefit–risk analysis

Meropenem
Merinfec® (AT), Meronem® (BE, CZ, DE, DK, ES, FI, GB, GR, HU, HR, NL, NO, PL, PT, SE, TR), Merrem® (IT)

Spectrum:
Very good in vitro activity against Gram-positive (non-methicillin-resistant *S. aureus* and *E. faecium*) and Gram-negative bacteria incl. *Pseudomonas* species (not *Stenotrophomonas maltophilia*)

Dosage:

• Adults and children >12 years	0.5–1 g i.v. q8h in meningitis: 2 g q8h
• Children (>3 months to 12 years)	30–60 mg/kg/day i.v. divided into 3 doses; in meningitis: 40 mg/kg q8h
In renal insufficiency (adults):	With CrCl of 50–26 ml/min, 0.5–1 g q12h; with CrCl of 25–10 ml/min, 0.25–0.5 g q12h; with CrCl <10 ml/min, 0.25–0.5 g q24h

In renal insufficiency (children):

CrCl	Dose (% of normal dose)
40	70 (divided into 2 doses)
20	40 (divided into 2 doses)
10	20 (single dose)
Anuria	15 (single dose)

Adverse effects:
Gastrointestinal symptoms, allergies, local reactions, exanthema, elevated transaminases, blood count changes, headaches

Contraindications:
Hypersensitivity

Remarks:
Monosubstance, additional cilastatin not necessary. Do not use in patients with known anaphylactic reaction to penicillins

Metronidazole
Alvidral® (GR), Amotein® (ES), Anaeromet® (BE), Clont® (DE), Deflamon® (IT), Dumozol® (PT), Efloran® (CZ, HR), Elyzol® (AT, DK, FI, FR, GB, NL, NO, SE)

Spectrum:
Anaerobes (*Bacteroides fragilis*, clostridia and anaerobic cocci), trichomonads, lambliae, amoebas

Dosage:

• Adults	400 mg p.o. q8–12h*; 500 mg i.v. q8–12h
• Children	20–30 mg/kg/day i.v. divided into 2 doses; 20–30 mg/kg/day p.o. divided into 2–3 doses
	*Dosages in formulations vary in different European countries. In Italy, for instance, dosages for the oral formulation is 250–500 mg only, recommended dosage for adults is 500 mg p.o. q6h, and 1 g i.v. q12h
In renal insufficiency (adults):	No significant prolongation of half-life. However, with serum creatinine 10 mg/dl and CrCl <10 ml/min only one dose (400 mg p.o.; 500 mg i.v.) q12h should be given. The duration of treatment should not exceed 10 days

In renal insufficiency (children):

CrCl	Dose (% of normal dose)
40	100 (divided into 3 doses)
20	100 (divided into 3 doses)
10	50 (divided into 2 doses)
Anuria	50 (divided into 2 doses)

Adverse effects:
Gastrointestinal symptoms, sensations of taste, neuropathy, leukopenia, headaches, ataxia; elevated transaminases, alcohol intolerance

Contraindications:
Hypersensitivity to metronidazole; in first 3 months of gestation only in life-threatening circumstances (from 4th month of pregnancy onward, after benefit–risk analysis)

Remarks:
In severe hepatic insufficiency, only after benefit–risk analysis; high sodium content of i.v. solution

---

Mezlocillin
Baypen® (AT, DE, FR, GB, IT, SE, TR)

Spectrum:
Gram-positive (not: β-lactamase-forming staphylococci, enterococci, listeriae) and Gram-negative bacteria, incl. *Ps. aeruginosa*; some anaerobes (*Bacteroides*, peptostreptococci)

Dosage:

• Adults	2–5 g i.v. q8h 2–3 g i.v. q8–12h in biliary tract or urinary tract infections
• Children 1–14 years	75 mg/kg i.v. q8h
• Infants >3 kg	75 mg/kg i.v. q8h
• Infants <3 kg; premature babies	75 mg/kg i.v. q12h
In renal insufficiency (adults):	With CrCl <10 ml/min, max. 5 g/day q12h

In renal insufficiency (children):

CrCl	Dose (% of normal dose)
40	100
20	50 (divided into 2 doses)
10	50 (divided into 2 doses)
Anuria	50 (single dose)

Adverse effects:
Hypersensitivity reactions, gastrointestinal symptoms, transiently elevated transaminases, eosinophilia, dysgeusia, leukocyte depression, hypokalaemia, thrombocytopenia, impaired coagulation, cramps (at very high dosage)

Contraindications:
Penicillin allergy

Remarks:
Together with piperacillin, penicillin of choice for life-threatening infections until the pathogen is identified. Dose reduction in severe liver disease

---

Micafungin
Mycamine® (DE, IT)

Spectrum:
Candida species (*C. albicans*, *C. glabrata*, *C. guilliermondii*, *C. krusei*, *C. parapsilosis* and *C. tropicalis*) including azole- and amphotericin B-resistant species, Aspergillus species. Standardized susceptibility testing methods have been proposed, but the correlation between the results of susceptibility studies and clinical outcome has not been established.

Dosage:

- Adults
Candidemia, disseminated candidiasis, candida peritonitis and abscess: 100 mg/day i.v.
In endocarditis and other cardiovascular infections dosage might be increased up to 150 mg/day i.v.
Esophageal candidiasis: 100 mg/day i.v.
Prophylaxis 50 mg/day i.v. (<40 kg: 1 mg/kg/day)
Loading dose not required. Infuse over 1 h

- Children and   100 mg/day i.v.
  adolescents
  (≥40 kg)

- Children (≤40 kg)   2 mg/kg/day i.v.

Adverse effects:
Nausea, vomiting, diarrhoea, pyrexia, headache, hypokalae-mia, thrombocytopenia, hemolysis, hemolytic anaemia, hae-moglobinuria, histamine-mediated symptoms (e.g. rash, pruri-tus, facial swelling, vasodilatation), hypersensitivity reactions, anaphylaxis and anaphylactoid reactions (including shock), abnormal liver function tests, renal dysfunction

Contraindications:
Hypersensitivity to micafungin, any component of drug, or other echinocandins

Remarks:
No dose adjustment in patients with renal impairment required. No supplementary dosing following to hemodialysis. No dose adjustment in patients with moderate hepatic impairment. Use in pregnancy only if potential benefits of treatment out-weigh potential foetal risk. Caution if administrated to a nursing mother.
Monitor of sirolimus, itraconazole or nifedipine toxicity, dosage reduction, if necessary

Minocycline
Logryx® (FR), Minocin® (AT, BE, ES, GB, GR, IT, PT), Mino-cyclin® (DE)

Spectrum:
Gram-positive and Gram-negative pathogens, mycoplasmas, chlamydiae, borreliae, *Coxiella burnetii*, not: *Proteus* species, *Ps. aeruginosa, Nocardia asteroides*; relatively frequent resist-ance in pneumococci, streptococci, staphylococci and Gram-negative bacteria

Dosage:

- Adults   initially 200 mg,
                                         then q12h 100 mg p.o.

- Children   initially 4 mg/kg,
  >8 years old   then q12h 2 mg/kg p.o.

In renal   With minocycline no dose reduction is
insufficiency   necessary in patients with renal insuffi-
(adults and   ciency. Discontinuation of minocycline
children):   should be considered only in extreme re-
                                         nal insufficiency

Adverse effects:
Gastrointestinal symptoms, exanthema, phototoxic reactions, rarely anaphylaxis, dental discoloration, hepatotoxicity, pseudotumor cerebri, negative nitrogen balance (raised urea nitrogen), relatively frequent vestibular phenomena (dizziness, ataxia 5–7%, more frequent in women, higher blood concentration than in men)

Contraindications:
Pregnancy; do not prescribe to children

Moxifloxacin
Actira® (AT, DE, ES), Avalox® (AT, BE, CZ, DE, DK, FI, GB, GR, HR, IT, NL, PL, PT, SE, TR), Izilox® (FR)

Spectrum:
Nearly all Gram-positive and Gram-negative pathogens and anaerobes; particularly effective against respiratory tract pathogens (pneumococci, *H. influenzae*, moraxellae, chlamydiae, mycoplasmas, legionellae), weak against *Ps. aeruginosa*

Dosage:

- Adults   400 mg p.o., i.v. q24h

In renal insufficiency: No dose adjustment necessary

Adverse effects:
Gastrointestinal symptoms, stupor, prolonged QT interval in patients with existing hypokalaemia or hypocalcaemia, dysgeusia, raised liver values, fulminant hepatitis, exanthema, Stevens–Johnson syndrome

Contraindications:
Pregnancy and lactation, children and adolescents, prolonged QT interval, previous symptomatic cardiac rhythm disturbances; restricted liver function or elevated transaminases because of absence of pharmacokinetic data

Remarks:
No interaction with theophylline, no photosensitisation, slight risk of resistance

---

Netilmicin
Certomycin® (AT), Netilin® (GB), Netrocin® (ES), Netromicina® (PT), Netromicine® (BE, CZ, FR, HR, NL, PL, TR), Netromycin® (GR), Nettacin® (IT), Netylin® (DK, FI, NO, SE)

Spectrum:
Gram-positive bacteria (staphylococci, not: pneumococci, streptococci, enterococci), Gram-negative bacteria, including most gentamicin- and tobramycin-resistant pathogens

Dosage:

• Adults	4–6 mg/kg/day i.m., i.v. simplified dosing scheme: 200 mg q12h or total dose once daily (same effect!) in life-threatening infections: up to 7.5 mg/kg/day
• Children >1 year old	6–7.5 mg/kg/day i.m., i.v. divided into 3 doses

| • Neonates | 6 mg/kg/day i.m., i.v. divided into 2 doses |
| • Neonates >1 week old | 7.5–9 mg/kg/day i.m., i.v. divided into 3 doses |

In renal insufficiency (adults):	CrCl	Max. dose (g)	DI (h)
	120	0.15	12
	45	0.1	12
	18	0.1	24
	8	0.05	24
	2	0.025	24
	0.5	0.025	24

In renal insufficiency (children):	CrCl	Dose (% of normal dose)
	40	60 (single dose); LD 5 mg/kg
	20	30 (single dose); LD 4 mg/kg
	10	15 (single dose); LD 3 mg/kg
	Anuria	10 (single dose) or 20 after HD; LD 2 mg/kg

Adverse effects:
Nephro- and ototoxicity, particularly if peak concentration >10 µg/ml (only with multiple dosing) or trough concentration >2 µg/ml (with single and multiple dosing), with previous aminoglycoside therapy or simultaneous administration of furosemide or ethacrynic acid. Eosinophilia, arthralgia, exanthema, fever, neuromuscular blockade

Contraindications:
Parenteral administration in first 3 months of pregnancy; from 4th month of gestation onward, only in life-threatening circumstances

Remarks:
Do not mix aminoglycoside solutions with penicillins or cephalosporins (inactivation of the aminoglycosides). Less ototoxic than other aminoglycosides

Nitrofurantoin
Furadantin® (AT, GB, IT, NO, SE), Furadantina® (PT), Fura-dantine® (BE, FR, NL), Furantoin® (CZ), Furantoina® (ES), Furedan® (IT), Furolin® (GR), Macrofuran® (FI), Nifurantin® (DE), Ninur® (HR), Piyeloseptyl® (TR), Siraliden® (PL)

Spectrum:
Staphylococci, streptococci, enterococci, *E. coli*, klebsiellae, *Enterobacter*

Dosage:

• Adults   100 mg p.o. q6–12h

In renal insufficiency: Contraindicated

Adverse effects:
Nausea, vomiting, pulmonary infiltrations, allergic pulmonary oedema, photosensitisation, neuropathy, headaches, dizziness, rarely leukopenia, anaemia, allergy

Contraindications:
Restricted liver function (CrCl <50 ml/min), pregnancy; do not use in neonates under 2 months

Remarks:
In severe liver diseases other antibiotics should be used

Norfloxacin
Alenbit® (GR), Amicrobin® (ES), Barazan® (DE), Chibroxol® (BE, NL, PT), Diperflox® (IT), Floxacin® (AT), Gyrablock® (CZ), Lexinor® (FI, SE), Noroxin® (ES, FR, GB, IT, NL, PT, TR), Zo-roxin® (AT, BE, DK)

Spectrum:
Nearly all Gram-positive and Gram-negative pathogens causing urinary tract infection and acute bacterial gastroenteritis

Dosage:

• Adults	400 mg p.o. q12h
In renal insufficiency:	With CrCl of <30 ml/min, corresponding to serum creatinine values of 2.5–5 mg/dl, the dose is 400 mg once daily

Adverse effects:
Loss of appetite, nausea, diarrhoea, allergy, dizziness, headaches, tendinitis, worsening of myasthenia gravis; very rarely leukopenia, eosinophilia, elevated transaminases, alkaline phosphatases and creatinine

Contraindications:
Pregnancy and lactation, epilepsy; do not prescribe to children and adolescents

Remarks:
Compared with other antibiotics, above average development of resistance in *Pseudomonas* and staphylococci. Dose reduction in severe liver disease

---

Nystatin
Fungicidin® (CZ), Fungostatin® (TR), Macmiror® (CZ, PL, TR), Moronal® (DE), Mycostatin® (AT, BE, DK, ES, FI, FR, GR, IT, NO, PT, SE), Nystan® (GB)

Spectrum:
Candida species, *Blastomyces* species, *Coccidioides immitis, Cryptococcus neoformans, Histoplasma capsulatum* and *Aspergillus* species; inactive against dermatophytes and actinomycetes

Dosage:

• Adults and children	1.5–3 million IU/day p.o. divided into 3 doses

• Infants	0.5–1 million IU/day p.o. divided into 3 doses
In renal insufficiency (adults and children):	No dose reduction necessary

Adverse effects:

Very rare, at high oral dosage retching, vomiting, loose stools, hypersensitivity reactions

Remarks:

The antimycotic for therapy and prophylaxis of intestinal yeast mycoses; practically no resorption

---

Ofloxacin
Docofloxacine® (BE), Oflocin® (IT), Tarivid® (DE)

Spectrum:

Nearly all Gram-positive and Gram-negative pathogens including *H. influenzae*, salmonellae, shigellae, *Yersinia, Campylobacter*, neisseriae, legionellae; not anaerobes. Only slight activity against *Ps. aeruginosa, Acinetobacter*, serratiae, enterococci, streptococci, pneumococci

Dosage:

• Adults	100–200 mg p.o., i.v. q12h, in severe infections: 200–400 mg p.o., i.v. q12h

In renal insufficiency:	CrCl ml/min	Maintenance dose mg/day
	50–20	100–200
	<20	100
	Haemo- or peritoneal dialysis	

Adverse effects:
Loss of appetite, nausea, diarrhoea, allergy, dizziness, headaches, skin lesions, CNS disturbances, psychoses, arthralgia and tendinopathy, very rarely leukopenia, eosinophilia, elevated transaminases, alkaline phosphatases and creatinine

Contraindications:
Pregnancy and lactation, CNS diseases (especially epilepsy); do not prescribe to children and adolescents

Remarks:
In children and adolescents, only in life-threatening circumstances. *Beware!* Development of resistance, particularly in *Pseudomonas* and staphylococci. Dose reduction in severe liver diseases

---

Oxacillin
Bristopen® (FR), InfectoStaph® (DE), Oxacillin® (CZ), Pentastapho® (BE, IT), Stapenor® (AT)

Spectrum:
Methicillin-susceptible staphylococci

Dosage:

• Adults	1(–2) g i.v. q6h (max. 12 g/day)
• Children 1–6 years	1–2 g/day i.v. divided into 4 doses
• Infants >3 months	80 mg/kg/day i.v. divided into 4 doses
• Infants	60 mg/kg/day i.v. divided into 3 doses
• Neonates and premature babies	40 mg/kg/day i.v. divided into 2 doses
In renal insufficiency (adults):	With CrCl <10 ml/min the daily dose should not exceed 1 g q6h (or 1 g q4h in endocarditis)

In renal insufficiency (children):	CrCl	Dose (% of normal dose)
	40	100 (divided into 4 doses)
	20	75 (divided into 4 doses)
	10	60 (divided into 3 doses)
	Anuria	30 (single dose)

Adverse effects:
Diarrhoea, fever, exanthema, elevated transaminases, Hb decrease, leukopenia. Rarely interstitial nephritis (haematuria), eosinophilia, cerebral cramps at very high dosage

Contraindications:
Penicillin allergy

Remarks:
Drug of choice for methicillin-susceptible *Staphylococcus aureus* (MSSA).
Dose reduction in restricted liver function

Penicillin G
Various preparations
Omnacilina® (PT), Penicillin Gruenenthal® (DE), Penidural® (GB, NL), Peniroger® (ES)

Spectrum:
Particularly meningococci, pneumococci, streptococci, gonococci

Dosage:

• Adults and children >12 years	Low dose: 0.6–1.2 million IU i.v. q6h. High dose: 4 million IU i.v. q4h (max. 60 million IU/day) (e.g. meningitis)
• Children >1 year old	50,000–500,000 IU/kg/day i.m., i.v. divided into 4–6 doses
• Neonates	50,000–100,000 IU/kg/day i.m., i.v. divided into 2 doses

• Neonates >4 weeks old	50,000–1 million IU/kg/day i.m., i.v. divided into 3–4 doses	

In renal insufficiency (adults):	CrCl	Max. dose (million IU)	DI (h)
	120	5	6
	45	5	8
	18	4	8
	8	5	12
	2	3	12
	0.5	2	12[8]

[8] Two to three haemodialyses per week are a necessary precondition. One normal dose initially

In renal insufficiency (children):	CrCl	Dose (% of normal dose)
	40	75 (divided into 3 doses)
	20	60 (divided into 3 doses)
	10	50 (divided into 2 doses)
	Anuria	20 (divided into 2 doses) or 30 after HD

Adverse effects:
Drug fever, exanthema, haemolytic anaemia, blood count changes, anaphylaxis (0.004–0.015%), cramps (only at high doses and with rapid i.v. injection, e.g. 5 million IU per 5 min), rarely interstitial nephritis

Contraindications:
Penicillin allergy

Remarks:
The sodium and potassium content of penicillin G is relevant in severe cardiac or renal insufficiency. Current pneumococcal resistance in Europe ▶ Chap. 7, (see: EARSS data on the website: http://www.rivm.nl/earss/) Conversion: 1 million IU Penicillin G = 600 mg

9

Penicillin V (phenoxymethylpenicillin)
Isocillin® (DE), Megacillin oral® (DE) and other in DE, Oracil-line® (FR), Phenoxymethylpenicillin® (GB)

Spectrum:
Particularly meningococci, pneumococci, streptococci, gonococci

Dosage:

• Adults and children >12 years	0.5–1.5 million IU p.o. q6–8h
• Children >4 months	40,000–60,000 (max. 160,000) IU/kg/day p.o. divided into 3–4 doses
• Children ≤4 months	40,000–60,000 IU/kg/day p.o. divided into 3 doses
In renal insufficiency (adults):	Up to CrCl of 30–15 ml/min, no dose reduction at a dosing interval of 8 h; with anuria, extend the interval to 12 h

In renal insufficiency (children):	CrCl	Dose (% of normal dose)
	40	100 (divided into 3 doses)
	20	100 (divided into 3 doses)
	10	50 (divided into 2 doses)
	Anuria	50 after HD

Adverse effects:
Drug fever, exanthema, gastrointestinal symptoms, haemolytic anaemia, anaphylaxis (0.004–0.015%)

Contraindications:
Penicillin allergy

Remarks:
Current pneumococcal resistance in Europe ► Chap. 7, (see: EARSS data on the website: http://www.rivm.nl/earss/). Another commercially available phenoxypenicillin derivative

is propicillin (Baycillin®). Conversion: 0.7 g propicillin = 1 million IU

Piperacillin
Avocin® (IT), Piperacillin® (DE), Piperilline® (FR), Piperital® (IT)
Pipraks® (TR), Pipril® (AT, CZ, ES, FI, GB, GR, HR, PT)

Spectrum:
Especially effective against *Pseudomonas, Proteus, E. coli.*
Partially effective against *Klebsiella, Enterobacter, Citrobacter, Bacteroides.* Not *S. aureus* (!)

Dosage:

- Adults   2–4 g i.v. q6–8h
- Children   100–300 mg/kg/day i.v. divided into 2–4
  >1 month   doses
- Neonates   150–300 mg/kg/day i.v. divided into 3
                  doses

In renal insufficiency (adults):	CrCl	Max. dose (g)	DI (h)
	120	4	6
	45	4	8
	18	4	8
	8	4	12
	2	4	12
	0.5	2	8[9]

[9] Two to three haemodialyses per week are a necessary precondition. One normal dose initially

In renal insufficiency (children):	CrCl	Dose (% of normal dose)
	40	60 (divided into 3 doses)
	20	40 (divided into 3 doses)
	10	25 (divided into 2 doses)
	Anuria	15 (single dose)

Adverse effects:
Gastrointestinal symptoms, exanthema, fever, rarely elevated transaminases, interstitial nephritis, blood count changes

Contraindications:
Penicillin allergy

Remarks:
Penicillin of choice for *Pseudomonas* infections. Piperacillin contains approximately 2 mmol of sodium/g of piperacillin

---

Piperacillin/Tazobactam
Tazobac® (DE), Tazocel® (ES), Tazocilline® (FR), Tazocin® (BE, DK, GB, HU, IT, NL, NO, PL, SE, TR)

Spectrum:
Gram-positive (not methicillin-resistant staphylococci and *E. faecium*) and Gram-negative bacteria, especially *Pseudomonas, Proteus, E. coli,* particularly β-lactamase formers and anaerobes

Dosage:

- Adults and chil-   4.5 g i.v. q8h
  dren >12 years

- Children   <40 kg: 112.5 mg/kg q8h;
  2–12 years   >40 kg: as for adults

In renal insufficiency (adults):	CrCl	Max. dose (g)	DI (h)
	120	4.5	8
	45	4.5	8
	18	4.5	12
	8	4.5	12
	2	4.5	12
	0.5	2.25	12

In renal	CrCl	Dose (% of normal dose)
insufficiency	40	60 (divided into 3 doses)
(children):	20	40 (divided into 3 doses)
	10	35 (divided into 3 doses)
	Anuria	33 (divided into 3 doses)

Adverse effects:
Gastrointestinal symptoms, exanthema, fever, rarely elevated transaminases, interstitial nephritis, tendency towards brain cramps at very high concentrations

Contraindications:
Penicillin allergy, pregnancy and lactation; do not prescribe to children <2 years

Remarks:
Piperacillin preparations contain approximately 2 mmol of sodium/g of piperacillin

---

Posaconazole
Noxafil® (AT, DE, DK, ES, FR, GB, IT, NO, SE)

Spectrum:
Salvage therapy in treatment-resistant *Aspergillus* species, *Candida* species and species of *Fusarium, Rhizomucor, Mucor* and *Rhizopus*

Dosage:

- Therapy-resistant invasive mycoses
  400 mg (10 ml) p.o. q12h

- Oropharyngeal candidosis
  200 mg (5 ml) p.o. on day 1, then 100 mg (2.5 ml) p.o. for 13 days

- Prophylaxis of invasive mycoses
  200 mg (5 ml) p.o. q8h (start a few days before expected onset of neutropenia and continue for 7 days after neutrophil count rises to over 500 cells/mm^3)

Adverse effects:
Headaches, nausea, vomiting, raised liver enzymes, rash

Contraindications:
Simultaneous use of ergot alkaloids; simultaneous use of CYP3A4 substrates or HMG-CoA reductase inhibitors (e.g. simvastatin, lovastatin and atorvastatin)

Remarks:
Posaconazole should be taken at mealtimes or, in patients who are not eating meals, together with a nutritional supplement to increase resorption and assure adequate exposure

---

Protionamide
Ektebin® (DE), Isoprodian® (AT), Promid® (TR), Tebeform® (HU) Trevintix® (GB)

Spectrum:
Mycobacterium tuberculosis and *M. kansasii*

Dosage:

• Adults	10–15 mg/kg/day p.o., max. 1,000 mg/day in 1–2 doses
• Children	7.5–15 mg/kg p.o., max. 500 mg/day
In renal insufficiency (adults):	No data as yet. Intermittent therapy (1,000 mg 2–3 times weekly) should be considered

In renal insufficiency (children):	CrCl	Dose (% of normal dose)
	40	100
	20	50
	10	25 (check blood level)
	Anuria	25 (check blood level)

Adverse effects:
Gastrointestinal symptoms (up to 50%), hepatotoxicity, neutropenia, hypothermia, hypoglycaemia (in diabetics). Rarely: peripheral neuropathy, cramps, exanthema, purpura, stomatitis, menstrual disturbances

Contraindications:
First 3 months of pregnancy, severe liver damage, epilepsy, psychoses, alcoholism

Remarks:
Monitor transaminases monthly

Pyrazinamide
Piraldina® (IT, TR), Pyrafat® (DE, AT), Tebrazid® (BE), Tisamid® (CZ, FI)

Spectrum:
Mycobacterium tuberculosis

Dosage:

• Adults and adolescents	20–30 mg/kg/day p.o. in 1 dose; <50 kg: max. 1.5 g, 51–75 kg: max. 2 g, >75 kg: max. 2.5 g
• Children	30 mg/kg/day
In renal insufficiency (adults):	Weight 50 kg: 3.5 g twice weekly or 2.5 g three times weekly

In renal insufficiency (children):

CrCl	Dose (% of normal dose)
40	100
20	75 (single dose)
10	50 (single dose)
Anuria	100 after HD three times weekly

Adverse effects:
Arthralgia, raised uric acid, liver damage, gastrointestinal symptoms, rarely photosensitivity

Contraindications:
Severe liver damage, gout

Remarks:
Close monitoring of liver function, starting before treatment; in patients with severe liver diseases, use other antibiotics
Established drug combinations for the treatment of tuberculosis are:
Rifampin + isoniazid + pyrazinamide: Rifater® (FR, IT, ES)

Quinupristin/Dalfopristin
Synercid® (AT, CZ, DE, ES, FR, GB, IT, PL)

Spectrum:
Staph. aureus (incl. MRSA, GISA), coagulase-negative staphylococci, *Strep. pneumoniae* (including penicillin-resistant strains), *Strep. pyogenes, M. catarrhalis, E. faecium* (incl. VRE; not *E. faecalis*), *C. jeikeium, N. gonorrhoeae, L. monocytogenes*

Dosage:

• Adults	7.5 mg/kg q8h
In renal insufficiency:	No dose adjustment necessary

Adverse effects:
Inflammation, pain, thrombophlebitis with peripheral venous access (not with central venous catheter, CVC), myalgia, arthralgia, gastrointestinal symptoms, raised bilirubin (total and conjugated) and transaminases

Contraindications:
Intolerance of streptogramin antibiotics, severe hepatic insufficiency

Remarks:

Dose reduction in hepatic insufficiency; insufficient data on dosing in children and neonates; administration via CVC in 5% glucose solution over 60 min; incompatible with NaCl solutions; inhibition of the CYP-P450-3A4 enzyme system

---

Rifabutin

Ansatipine® (ES, FI, FR, SE), Mycobutin® (AT, BE, CZ, DE, GB, GR, IT, NL, PT, TR)

Spectrum:

Mycobacterium tuberculosis (incl. over 30% of rifampin-resistant strains), *M. leprae, M. avium-intracellulare, M. fortuitum, M. kansasii, M. marinum, M. ulcerans*

Dosage:

• Adults	Prophylaxis of MAC* infection: 0.3 g/day p.o. Therapy of MAC infection: 0.45–0.6 g/day p.o. (in combination with clarithromycin: 0.3 g/day p.o.) Therapy of (multiresistant) TB: 0.15 g/day p.o. (always combination therapy; in pre-treated patients 0.3–0.45 g/day p.o.) * MAC: *M. avium intracellulare* complex
In renal insufficiency:	With CrCl <30 ml/min, dose reduction by 50%

Adverse effects:

Gastrointestinal symptoms, elevated transaminases, leukopenia, thrombocytopenia, anaemia, joint and muscle pains, fever, erythema, rarely skin discoloration, orange colouring of the urine, hypersensitivity reactions (eosinophilia, bronchospasm, shock), mild to severe uveitis (reversible); increased risk of uveitis in combination with clarithromycin or fluconazole

Contraindications:
Hypersensitivity to rifabutin or rifampin, pregnancy, lactation, severe liver disease; do not combine with rifampin

Remarks:
Regular monitoring of leukocyte and thrombocyte counts and liver enzymes during treatment; drug-to-drug interactions with HAART (highly active anti-retroviral therapy) must be carefully evaluated

---

Rifampin/Rifampicin
Arficin® (CZ, HR), Eremfat® (AT, DE), Rifadin® (GB, GR, IT, NL, PT, SE, TR), Rifarm® (FI), Rimactan® (BE, DK, ES, FR, NO, SE), Tubocin® (HU)

Spectrum:
Mycobacterium tuberculosis, M. bovis, M. avium-intracellulare, M. leprae, M. kansasii, M. marinum; Gram-positive cocci, legionellae, chlamydiae, meningococci, gonococci, *H. influenzae;* not *M. fortuitum*

Dosage:

• Adults	600 mg p.o., i.v. q24h over 50 kg 450 mg p.o., i.v. q24h up to 50 kg
• Children	10–15 mg/kg/day p.o., i.v. in 1(–2) dose(s)
In renal insufficiency (adults and children):	Rifampin is not nephrotoxic and can be given in normal dosage (10 mg/kg, maximum dose 600 mg/day) in patients with various degrees of renal insufficiency

Adverse effects:
Gastrointestinal symptoms, drug fever, itching with or without rash, elevated transaminases and alkaline phosphatases, rarely jaundice, eosinophilia, CNS symptoms, thrombocytopenia, leukopenia

Contraindications:
Severe liver damage, jaundice; hypersensitivity to rifamycins

Remarks:
Monitoring of liver function, blood count and serum creatinine before and during treatment; no monotherapy owing to development of resistance. Multiple drug to drug interactions.
Established drug combinations for the treatment of tuberculosis are
Rifampin + isoniazid: Rifinah® (DE, FR, GB, GR, IT, NL, PT, TR), Rifamazid® (PL), Rimactazid® (DK, NO, SE)
Rifampin + isoniazid + pyrazinamide: Rifater® (AT, DE, ES, FR, IT, PT, TR), Rimcure® (NO, SE)
Rifampin + isoniazid + pyrazinamide + ethambutol: Rimstar® (DK)

Roxithromycin
Acevor® (GB, GR), Roxithromycin® (DE), Rulid® (BE, CZ, FR, GR, IT, PL, TR), Rulide® (AT, ES, NL, PT), Surlid® (DK, FI, SE)

Spectrum:
Gram-positive pathogens, particularly staphylococci, streptococci, pneumococci, *Corynebacterium diphtheriae,* mycoplasmas, *B. pertussis,* legionellae, chlamydiae, *Campylobacter,* relatively frequently resistant staphylococci

Dosage:

• Adults	150 mg p.o. q12h or 300 mg p.o. q24h
• Children	5–7.5 mg/kg/day p.o. divided into 2 doses
In renal insufficiency (adults and children):	No dose reduction necessary in the case of restricted renal function

Adverse effects:
Gastrointestinal symptoms, rarely exanthema, elevated transaminases

Contraindications:
Hypersensitivity to macrolides; accurate diagnosis imperative in QT-interval prolongation, hypokalaemia, hypomagnesaemia, bradycardia, cardiac insufficiency, cardiac dysrhythmia, simultaneous administration of QT-interval prolonging agents

Remarks:
Better pharmacokinetics than erythromycin; cut daily dose by half in severe liver dysfunction

---

Streptomycin
Estreptomicina® (ES), Pan-Streptomycin® (GR), Strep-Deva® (TR), Streptomicina® (IT), Streptomycin® (DE)

Spectrum:
M. tuberculosis, brucellae, *Yersinia pestis, Francisella tularensis,* staphylococci, enterococci, streptococci; not atypical mycobacteria

Dosage

- Adults   15 mg/kg/day i.v., i.m.
- Children   20–30 mg/kg/day i.v., i.m. divided into
  >6 months   2 doses
- Children   10–25 mg/kg/day i.v., i.m.

In renal insufficiency (adults):	CrCl	Max. dose (mg/kg)	DI (h)
	50–80	7.5	24
	10–50	7.5	48
	<10	7.5	72

Initial dose 15 mg/kg.
Additional dose after HD: 5 mg/kg

In renal	CrCl	Dose (% of normal dose)
insufficiency	40	80 (DI prolonged)
(children):	20	40 (DI prolonged)
	10	30 (DI prolonged)
	Anuria	25 (DI prolonged)

Adverse effects:
Dizziness, paraesthesias, nausea, vomiting, respiratory depression, visual impairment, nephrotoxicity, peripheral neuropathy, allergic cutaneous phenomena (ca. 5%), drug fever, leukopenia, ototoxicity, totally ca. 8%

Contraindications:
Pregnancy and lactation, premature babies and neonates; in advanced renal insufficiency only in life-threatening circumstances

Remarks:
Monthly audiogram. Do not combine streptomycin with other aminoglycosides or with rapid-acting diuretics such as ethacrynic acid and furosemide. In the treatment of tuberculosis the daily doses are administered all at once

---

Sulbactam
Betamaze® (FR), Combactam® (AT, DE)

Spectrum:
Inhibits β-lactamases of various Gram-positive and Gram-negative pathogens; intrinsic activity against *Acinetobacter baumanii*

Dosage:

- Adults   0.5–1 g i.v., i.m. at time of administration of antibiotic given in combination (max. 4 g/day)

• Children	50 mg/kg/day, divided according to dosing interval of antibiotic given in combination (max. 80 mg/kg/day)	

In renal insufficiency (adults):

CrCl	Max. dose (g)	DI (h)
30–15	1	12
15–5	1	24
<5	1	48

Additionally 1 g after HD

In renal insufficiency (children):

CrCl	Dose (% of normal dose)
40	60 (divided into 3 doses)
20	30 (divided into 2 doses)
10	20 (single dose)
Anuria	15 (single dose)

Adverse effects:
Allergic reactions, possibly even anaphylactic shock; blood count changes, gastrointestinal symptoms, rarely raised creatinine and transaminases, very rarely cramps, dizziness, headaches

Contraindications:
Allergies to β-lactam antibiotics, pregnancy and lactation (painstaking benefit–risk analysis)

Remarks:
Licensed for use in combination with mezlocillin, piperacillin, penicillin G and cefotaxime. Very good synergism for *Acinetobacter baumanii, Citrobacter,* staphylococci and anaerobes, moderate for *E. coli* and klebsiellae, very slight for *Ps. aeruginosa;* do not combine with piperacillin if CrCl <40 ml/min

Teicoplanin
Targocid® (AT, BE, CZ, DE, DK, ES, FI, FR, GB, GR, HR, NL, NO, PL, SE, TR), Targosid® (IT, PT)

Spectrum:
Particularly methicillin-resistant staphylococci (MRSA), enterococci, streptococci, *Clostridium difficile*, *Corynebacterium jeikeium*

Dosage:

• Adults	400 mg i.m. or i.v. q24h as brief infusion or injection (6 mg/kg/day); in severe infection: 800 mg q24h initially (12 mg/kg/day), in life-threatening infections: 3 doses of 800 mg each at intervals of 12 h, then 400 mg daily
• Children	first 3 doses at intervals of 12 h, 10 mg/kg i.v. each time, then 6–10 mg/kg/day i.v. as single dose
• Neonates <2 months	first dose 16 mg/kg/day i.v., then 8 mg/kg/day i.v. as single dose
In renal insufficiency (adults):	From the 4th day of treatment, dosage as follows: with CrCl 40–60 ml/min, ½ daily dose; with CrCl <40 ml/min: (CrCl/normal CrCl) × normal daily dose; with haemodialysis, 800 mg in 1st week, then 400 mg on day 8, day 15 etc.

In renal insufficiency (children):

CrCl	Dose (% of normal dose)
40	40 (single dose)
20	20 (single dose)
10	10 (single dose)
Anuria	LD 15 mg/kg, then depending on concentration

Adverse effects:
Less nephrotoxicity and flush than with vancomycin; elevated transaminases, alkaline phosphatases and serum creatinine; gastrointestinal symptoms

Contraindications:
Hypersensitivity to glycopeptides

Remarks:
The glycopeptide resistance of enterococci is genetically determined and exhibits three phenotypically different forms:
vanA: resistance to vancomycin and teicoplanin
vanB: vancomycin resistance, sensitive to teicoplanin
vanC: low-level vancomycin resistance (MIC 8–16 µg/ml), sensitive to teicoplanin

---

Telithromycin
Ketek® (AT, BE, DE, ES, FI, FR, GB, HR, IT, NO, PL, PT, SE)

Spectrum:
Staph. aureus, streptococci, *Strep. pneumoniae* (incl. macrolide- and penicillin-resistant strains), enterococci, *M. catarrhalis, B. pertussis*, mycoplasmas, chlamydiae, legionellae; weak action against *H. influenzae*; not: enterobacteria, *Pseudomonas, Acinetobacter*

Dosage:

• Adults and children >12 years	800 mg p.o. q24h
In renal insufficiency:	No dose adjustment necessary in slightly or moderately restricted renal function; with CrCl <30 ml/min, reduce alternate doses by half

Adverse effects:
Gastrointestinal symptoms, rarely allergies, eosinophilia, atrial arrhythmia, hypotonia, bradycardia, hepatitis

Contraindications:
Hypersensitivity to telithromycin; congenital QT syndrome; statins should be discontinued during telithromycin treatment; patients with myasthenia gravis display hepatitis after telithromycin therapy

Remarks:
First member of a new group of substances (ketolides) with a novel mechanism of action that may be characterised by low development of resistance

---

Tetracycline
Chropicyclin® (GR), Ciclobiotico® (PT), Tetracyclin® (DE), Tetralysal® (AT, BE, CZ, DK, ES, FI, FR, GB, IT, NO, PL, SE), Tetrarco® (NL)

Spectrum:
Gram-positive and Gram-negative pathogens, mycoplasmas, chlamydiae, not: *Proteus* species, *Ps. aeruginosa*; relatively frequent resistance in pneumococci, streptococci, staphylococci and Gram-negative bacteria

Dosage:

• Adults	0.5 g p.o. q6–12h
• Children >8 years old	25–50 mg/kg/day p.o. divided into 2–4 doses
In renal insufficiency:	The classic tetracyclines should no longer be used in renal insufficiency, as they can lead to increased urea concentration, vomiting and diarrhoea

Adverse effects:
Gastrointestinal symptoms, photosensitivity, exanthema, rarely anaphylaxis, dental discoloration, hepatotoxicity, pseudotumor cerebri, negative nitrogen balance (raised urea nitrogen)

Contraindications:
Pregnancy and lactation; do not prescribe to children

Tigecycline
Tygacil® (AT, CZ, DE, ES, FR, GB, IT, NO, SE)

Spectrum:
Gram-positive and Gram-negative pathogens incl. MRSA, VRE, ESBL; anaerobes; atypical pathogens; moderately effective against *Morganella* and *Proteus* species

Dosage:

• Adults	100 mg q24h as LD, then 50 mg q12h (infusion over 30–60 min)
• Children	No experience
In renal insufficiency:	No dose adjustment necessary
In hepatic in sufficiency Child Pugh C:	100 mg q24h as LD, then 25 mg q12h

Adverse effects:
Nausea, vomiting, diarrhoea, pancreatitis

Contraindications:
Known hypersensitivity to tigecycline

Remarks:
An increase in all-cause mortality has been observed in tigecycline-treated patients versus comparator-treated patients (reason unknown).
Risk of foetal harm during pregnancy.
Permanent discoloration of the teeth if administered during teeth development.

Tobramycin
Bramicil® (IT), Bramitob® (GB, NL), Brulamycin® (AT, CZ, HU), Distobram® (PT), Gernebcin® (DE), Nebcin® (HR, TR), Nebcina® (DK, FI, NO, SE), Nebcine® (FR), Obracin® (BE), TOBI® (DE, FR, GB, PL)

Spectrum:
Gram-positive pathogens (staphylococci, not: pneumococci, streptococci, enterococci, neisseriae), Gram-negative pathogens, particularly effective against *Ps. aeruginosa*

Dosage:

• Adults	3–6 mg/kg/day i.m., i.v. divided into 1–3 doses (30–60 min brief infusion)
• Children >1 year old	6–7.5 mg/kg/day i.m., i.v. divided into 3(–4) doses
• Neonates	5 mg/kg/day i.m., i.v. divided into 2 doses (also for body weight under 1,200 g)
• Neonates >4 weeks old	4.5–7.5 mg/kg/day i.m., i.v. divided into 3 doses

In renal insufficiency (adults):

CrCl	Max. dose (g)	DI (h)
120	0.12	8
45	0.12	12
18	0.04	12
8	0.04	24
2	0.02	24[10]
0.5	0.02	24[10, 11]

[10] In life-threatening cases, initial dose of 100 mg

[11] Two to three haemodialyses per week are considered necessary. One normal dose initially

In renal insufficiency (children):	CrCl	Dose (% of normal dose)
	40	60 (single dose); LD 4 mg/kg
	20	20 (single dose); LD 4 mg/kg
	10	10 (single dose); LD 3 mg/kg
	Anuria	5 (single dose) or 15 after HD; LD 2 mg/kg

Adverse effects:
Ototoxicity and nephrotoxicity, especially with peak concentrations >10 µg/ml or trough concentrations >2 µg/ml, with previous aminoglycoside therapy and with simultaneous administration of furosemide or ethacrynic acid. Eosinophilia, arthralgia, fever, exanthema; elevated transaminases

Contraindications:
Pregnancy and lactation; advanced renal insufficiency, preexisting labyrinthine deafness

Remarks:
Aminoglycoside of choice for *Ps. aeruginosa*. Do not mix aminoglycoside solutions with penicillins or cephalosporins (inactivation of the aminoglycosides); in patients with mucoviscidosis 8–10 mg/kg/day may be necessary; if appropriate, inhalation therapy with 80–160 mg q12h

---

Vancomycin
Diatracin® (ES), Edicin® (CZ, HR, HU, PL), Orivan® (FI), Vancocin® (AT, BE, GB, NL, PL, SE, TR), Vancocina® (IT)

Spectrum:
Particularly methicillin-resistant staphylococci, enterococci, *Clostridium difficile, Corynebacterium jeikeium*

Dosage:

- Adults

1 g i.v. q12h or 0.5 g q6h (never more than 10 mg/min, over at least 60 min)
125 mg p.o. q6h for *C. difficile* diarrhoea

- Children
  >1 year old

40 mg/kg/day i.v. divided into 2–4 doses

- Neonates

20 mg/kg/day i.v. divided into 2 doses (also for body weight under 1,200 g)

- Neonates
  >1 week old

30 mg/kg/day i.v. divided into 3 doses

In renal insufficiency (adults):

CrCl	Max. dose (g)	DI (h)
45	0.66	24
18	0.2	24
8	0.1	24

In anuric patients the initial dose is 15 mg/kg, the maintenance dose 1.9 mg/kg daily. In the case of regular haemodialysis the initial dose is normally 1 g, the maintenance dose 1 g weekly. Regular measurement of serum concentration is urgently recommended. Target levels: peak 20–50 µg/ml, trough 5–10 µg/ml

In renal insufficiency (children):

CrCl	Dose (% of normal dose)
40	30
20	10 (single dose)
10	5 (single dose)
Anuria	LD 15 mg/kg (then according to concentration)

Adverse effects:
Exanthema, anaphylactoid reactions, phlebitis, nephro- and ototoxicity, leukopenia, eosinophilia, thrombocytopenia, gastrointestinal symptoms

Contraindications:
Hypersensitivity to glycopeptides; in acute anuria and previous damage to the cochlear apparatus, only in life-threatening circumstances

Remarks:
Peak concentrations should not exceed 40 mg/l, trough concentrations should lie between 5 and 10 mg/l. Increased care with simultaneous administration of aminoglycosides and other potentially oto- and nephrotoxic substances. The glycopeptide resistance of enterococci is genetically determined and exhibits three phenotypically different forms:
vanA: resistance to vancomycin and teicoplanin
vanB: vancomycin resistance, sensitive to teicoplanin
vanC: low-level vancomycin resistance (MIC 8–16 µg/ml), sensitive to teicoplanin

---

Voriconazole
Vfend® (AT, BE, DE, CZ, DK, ES, FI, GB, IT, NL, NO, PL, PT, SE)

Spectrum:
Aspergillus species, numerous other filamentous fungi; *Candida* species, including some strains resistant to itraconazole and fluconazole; no effect in mucormycoses

Dosage i.v.:

• Adults	Day 1, 6 mg/kg i.v. q12h; from day 2, 4 mg/kg i.v.
• Children (2–12 years)	7 mg/kg q12h

Dosage p.o.:

• Adults >40 kg	Day 1, 400 mg p.o. q12h; from day 2, 200 mg p.o. q12h

- Adults <40 kg   Day 1, 200 mg p.o. q12h;
                      from day 2, 100 mg p.o. q12h

- Children   200 mg p.o. q12h
  (2–12 years)

**In renal   With CrCl <50 ml/min there is accumula-
insufficiency:**   tion of the carrier medium β-cyclodextrin,
                      so voriconazole should be given orally; in
                      the case of further i.v. therapy, serum
                      creatinine must be checked at frequent
                      intervals

Adverse effects:
Gastrointestinal symptoms, reversible increase in liver enzymes, rash; fairly frequently short-term and reversible functional visual impairments (blurred vision, increased light sensitivity), rarely anaphylaxis

Contraindications:
Administration of rifampin, carbamazepine, phenobarbital, ergot alkaloids, sirolimus, terfenadine, astemizole, cisapride, pimozide, quinidine; pregnancy and lactation; intolerance of voriconazole and other ingredients; with simultaneous administration of voriconazole and cytochrome P450 substrates, it may in occasional cases be necessary to adapt the dose of the former or the latter

Remarks:
Bioavailability >90%; good access to cerebrospinal fluid, can be used in cerebral aspergillosis; maximal infusion rate 3 mg/kg/h

Daily Treatment Costs

Parenteral antibiotic	Dosage	Daily treatment costs[12]
Amikacin	1 g q24h	**
Ampicillin	5 g q8h	*
Ampicillin/sulbactam	3 g q8h	*
Benzylpenicillin	5 million IU q6h	*
Cefazolin	1 g q12h	*
Cefepime	2 g q12h	**
Cefotaxime	2 g q8h	**
Cefotiam	2 g q8h	**
Ceftazidime	2 g q8h	***
Ceftriaxone	2 g q24h	**
Cefuroxime	1.5 g q6h	*
Ciprofloxacin	400 mg q8h	***
Clarithromycin	500 mg q12h	**
Clindamycin	600 mg q8h	**
Daptomycin	350 mg q24h	***
Doripenem	500 mg q8h	**
Doxycycline	100 mg q12h	*
Ertapenem	1 g q24h	**
Erythromycin	1 g q12h	**
Flucloxacillin	4 g q8h	**
Fosfomycin	5 g q8h	**
Gentamicin	80 mg q8h	*
Imipenem	1 g q8h	***
Levofloxacin	750 mg q24h	**
Linezolid	600 mg q12h	***

Parenteral antibiotic	Dosage	Daily treatment costs[12]
Meropenem	1 g q8h	***
Metronidazole	500 mg q8h	*
Mezlocillin	3 g q8h	**
Moxifloxacin	400 mg q24h	**
Piperacillin	4 g q8h	**
Piperacillin/tazobactam	4.5 g q8h	**
Quinupristin/dalfopristin	0.5 g q8h	****
Rifampin	600 mg q24h	*
Teicoplanin	400 mg q24h	***
Tigecycline	50 mg q12h	***
Tobramycin	240 mg q24h	*
Cotrimoxazole	960 mg q12h	*
Vancomycin	1 g q12h	**

[12] Pharmacy sales price in €

Antimycotic	Dosage	Daily treatment costs[13]
Amphotericin B	50 mg q24h	**
Amphotericin B liposomal	200 mg q24h	*****
Anidulafungin i.v.	100 mg q24h	*****
Caspofungin	50 mg q24h	****
Fluconazole i.v.	400 mg q24h	**
Fluconazole p.o.	200 mg q24h	*
Flucytosine	2500 mg q6h	****
Itraconazole i.v.	200 mg q12h	***
Itraconazole p.o.	200 mg q12h	*
Micafungin i.v.	100 mg q24h	*****
Voriconazole i.v.	300 mg q12h	*****
Voriconazole p.o.	200 mg q12h	***
Posaconazole i.v.	400 mg q12h	***
Posaconazole p.o.	100 mg q24h	*

* ≤ 50 €
** ≤100 €
*** ≤200 €
**** ≤400 €
***** ≤800 €
[13] Pharmacy sales price category

10 Antibiotic Therapy of the Principal Infections in Children and Adults

Antibiotic dosages are given only if they differ from the recommendations in Chap. 9.

Actinomycosis

Pathogens:
Actinomyces species (principally *A. israelii*)

Primary Therapy:
Penicillin G 10–20 IU/day or ampicillin 50 mg/kg/day i.v. 4–6 weeks, then penicillin V 2–4 g/day or amoxicillin 500 mg p.o. q8h

Alternatives:
Doxycycline, clindamycin, ceftriaxone; in penicillin allergy/pregnancy: erythromycin, roxithromycin

Remarks:
Surgical intervention is frequently necessary. Treatment duration 3–6 months for thoracic or abdominal actinomycoses; 3–6 weeks for cervicofacial forms

Amebiasis

Pathogen:
Entamoeba histolytica (not *E. dispar*)

Therapy (intestinal form):
Metronidazole 500–750 mg p.o. q8h for 10 days, then paromomycin 500 mg p.o. q8h for 10 days

Remarks:
Owing to the danger of tissue invasion, asymptomatic excreters of *E. histolytica* should also be treated (with paromomycin only, 500 mg p.o. q8h for 7 days); intestinal lumen amebicide to prevent recurrence. In severe or extraintestinal infections (e.g. liver abscess): start with metronidazole i.v. for 10 days, then paromomycin for 7 days. In case of abscess greater than 3 cm, surgical aspiration might be required.

Amnionitis, Septic Abortion

Most Frequent Pathogens:
Bacteroides and other anaerobic bacteria, group A and B streptococci, enterobacteria, *C. trachomatis*

Primary Therapy:
Ampicillin/sulbactam + doxycycline (see remarks)

Alternatives:
Cephalosporins (3rd gen.) + clindamycin, ertapenem + doxycycline

Remarks:
Doxycycline is contraindicated in pregnancy

Arthritis

Most Frequent Pathogens:
- Adults: *S. aureus*, gonococci, *Kingella kingae*; after surgery or joint puncture: *S. epidermidis* (40%), *S. aureus* (20%), streptococci, *Pseudomonas*
  Chronic monarthritis: brucellae, mycobacteria, nocardiae, fungi
  After foreign body implantation: *S. aureus, S. epidermidis*
- Children (without osteomyelitis): *S. aureus*, group A streptococci, pneumococci, *Kingella kingae*, *H. influenzae*, other Gram-negative bacteria

- Infants: *S. aureus*, enterobacteria, group B streptococci, gonococci

Primary Therapy:
- Adults: oxacillin or flucloxacillin + cephalosporin (3rd gen.)
  After joint puncture: vancomycin + cephalosporin (3rd gen.)
  Chronic monarthritis: according to pathogen
- Children and infants: oxacillin or flucloxacillin + cephalosporin (3rd gen.)

Alternatives:
- Adults: oxacillin or flucloxacillin + ciprofloxacin
- Children and infants: oxacillin or flucloxacillin + aminoglycoside

Remarks:
Gram staining and methylene blue staining of pus and of blood cultures usually provide important clues to the pathogen. Surgical consultation and sometimes intervention is necessary. If MRSA rate high: vancomycin instead of oxacillin/flucloxacillin. Intra-articular instillation of antibiotics is not recommended. Treatment duration (2–)3 weeks in adults, (3–)4 weeks in children and infants; 4–6 weeks in infections of prostheses. For monoarticular arthritis: if Gram-stain suggests *S. aureus*: oxacillin/flucloxacillin or 2nd generation cephalosporin; if Gram-stain is negative: 3rd generation cephalosporin, e.g. ceftriaxone, cefotaxime, ceftizoxime. For gonococcal arthritis: ceftriaxone 1 g for 7–10 days.

Aspergillosis

Pathogens:
Aspergillus species

Primary Therapy:
- Adults:
  Voriconazole (6 mg/kg i.v. q12h on day 1, then 4 mg/kg i.v. q12h or 200 mg p.o. q12h if BW =40 kg, 100 mg p.o. q12h if BW <40 kg)
- Children:
  Voriconazole (5 mg/kg i.v. q12h);
  Caspofungin (50 mg/m2 /day);
  Liposomal amphotericin B 3–5 mg/kg/day;
  Micafungin 100–150 mg/day i.v.;
  Posaconazole 200 mg p.o. q6h until stabilization of disease, then 400 mg p.o. q12h;

Alternatives:
Caspofungin (70 mg i.v. on day 1, then 50 mg/day i.v.); Posaconazole (10 ml p.o. q12h)

Remarks:
Combination therapy not recommended – limited experience with anidulafungin and posaconazole in children.

Bacteriuria (Asymptomatic)

Most Frequent Pathogens:
Various pathogens, mostly Gram-negative

Primary Therapy:
Antibiotics not indicated [exceptions: pregnancy, immune suppression before and after urologic surgery (because of obstruction); therapy based on culture and antibiogram]

Borreliosis (Lyme Disease)

Pathogen:
Borrelia burgdorferi

Therapy:
Erythema migrans, facial palsy
- Adults: doxycycline 100 mg p.o. q12h or ampicillin 500 mg p.o. q8h or cefuroxime axetil 500 mg p.o. q12h or erythromycin 250 mg p.o. q6h, each for 14 days
- Children: amoxicillin 50 mg/kg/day p.o. in 3 doses or cefuroxime axetil 30 mg/kg/day p.o. in 2 doses or erythromycin 30 mg/kg/day p.o. in 3 doses, each for 14–21 days

Carditis (p.o. in AV block I, otherwise i.v.)
- Adults: ceftriaxone 2 g i.v. q24h or penicillin G 24 million IU/day i.v. or doxycycline 100 mg p.o. q12h or amoxicillin 250–500 mg p.o. q8h, each for 14–21 days
- Children: ceftriaxone 75–100 mg/kg/day i.v. in 1 dose or penicillin G 300,000 IU/kg/day i.v. in 4–6 doses or amoxicillin 50 mg/kg/day p.o. in 3 doses, each for 14–21 days

Meningitis, encephalitis
- Adults: ceftriaxone 1–2 g i.v. or penicillin G 20 million IU/day i.v., each for 14–28 days
- Children: ceftriaxone 100 mg/kg/day i.v. in 1 dose or penicillin G 300,000 IU/day in 4–6 doses, each for 14–28 days

Arthritis
- i.v. therapy as for meningitis or p.o. therapy (for 30–60 days) with doxycycline or amoxicillin or ceftriaxone 2 g i.v. q24h for 15–21 days

Remarks:
Antibiotic therapy in the early phase (inflamed tick bite, erythema chronicum migrans) can prevent late complications. A single dose of 200 mg doxycycline after tick bite may prevent borreliosis, but prophylaxis seems justified only in particular situations (satiated ticks in place for ≥24 h, highly endemic areas). In the early phase serology is often negative, so in the

case of clinical suspicion it should be repeated 2 weeks later; institute treatment if clinical suspicion coincides with positive serology (raised IgM titre). No therapy in asymptomatic sero-positivity.

10

Brain Abscess

Most Frequent Pathogens:
Acute: streptococci (up to 70%), *Bacteroides, S. aureus*, anaerobic cocci, Enterobacteria
Postoperative, posttraumatic: *S. aureus*, enterobacteria

Primary Therapy:

Frontal lobes dentogenic, sinusitis	Penicillin G + metronidazole or cefotaxime + metronidazole or ceftriaxone + metronidazole
Temporal lobes, cerebellum otogenic	Penicillin G + metronidazole + ceftazidime
Multiple brain abscesses, metastatic	Oxacillin or flucloxacillin + metronidazole + cefotaxime or ceftriaxone
Postoperative	Ceftazidime + vancomycin or teicoplanin
Brain abscess after penetrating trauma	Cefotaxime + oxacillin or flucloxacillin

Remarks:
Surgical consultation and possible intervention necessary. Duration of treatment 4–8 weeks. Antibiotic dosages (daily doses i.v.): penicillin G up to 24 million IU, metronidazole 500 mg q6h, cefotaxime 1–2 g q4–8h, maximum dose 12 g, ceftazidime 2g q6h, ceftriaxone 2g q12h, flucloxacillin 4 g q8h, vancomycin 1 g q12h; teicoplanin initially 800 mg, from day 2: 400 mg. In staphylococcal ventriculitis and external CSF drainage, pos-

sibly vancomycin 10 mg intraventricularly once daily. In nocardiosis: cotrimoxazole, minocycline or imipenem/cilastatin

Bronchitis

Most Frequent Pathogens:
Acute bronchitis: mostly viruses
Chronic bronchitis (acute exacerbation): viruses in up to 50% of cases; pneumococci, streptococci, *H. influenzae, Moraxella catarrhalis, Mycoplasma pneumoniae*

Therapy:
- Adults:
  Acute bronchitis (viruses): no antibiotic therapy necessary;
  Chronic severe bronchitis (acute exacerbation): amoxicillin/clavulanic acid, ampicillin/sulbactam, azithromycin, clarithromycin, quinolone (group IV); 5–10 days
  Bronchiectasis: an antibiotic active against *Pseudomonas*
- Children: oral penicillins, oral cephalosporins, erythromycin; 7 days (chemotherapy frequently superfluous due to mainly viral genesis)
- Infants: chemotherapy (penicillins) necessary only in otitis media and bronchial pneumonia, 7 days; mostly viral genesis

Remarks:
Clinical trials show variable results with antibiotics for chronic bronchitis. Patients with moderate to severe episodes (FEV <50%) do benefit. If cough persists for >14 days, consider *Bordetella pertussis* (also in adults). Penicillin resistance of pneumococci at MIC =2 mg/l; partial resistance at MIC >0.125 mg/l. In both cases cefotaxime, ceftazidime, ceftriaxone, quinolones (groups III, IV), telithromycin. Current resistance rates of pneumococci vary in different European countries ► Chap. 7.

Brucellosis

Most Frequent Pathogens:
Brucella abortus (Bang disease), *B. melitensis* (Malta fever)

Primary Therapy:
- Adults and children >8 years of age: 600–900 mg/day rifampin p.o. or
  gentamicin 2 mg/kg i.v. q8h for 7 days + 100 mg doxycycline p.o. q12h for 6 weeks
- Children <8 years of age: 5 mg/kg cotrimoxazole i.v. q12h for 6 weeks + gentamicin 2 mg/kg i.v. q8h for 2 weeks

Alternatives:
- Adults and children >8 years of age: 100 mg doxycycline q12h for 6 weeks + 1 g streptomycin i.m. for 2 weeks; TMP-SMX 4 × 1 DS × 6 weeks + gentamicin × 2–3 weeks

Candidiasis

Pathogens:
Candida species

Therapy:
- Skin: amphotericin B, clotrimazole, miconazole, nystatin locally q6–8h times daily for 7–14 days
- Thrush: oral nystatin or fluconazole 100–200 mg p.o.
- Esophagitis: fluconazole 200–400 mg p.o.; for fluconazole non-responding patients itraconazole 200 mg p.o., posaconazole 400 mg p.o., voriconazole 200 mg p.o. q12h or amphotericin B oral suspension or caspofungin 70 mg i.v. day 1, then 50 mg i.v. or anidulafungin 100 mg i.v. day 1, then 50 mg i.v. or micafungin 100 mg i.v.
- Urinary tract: generally catheter colonisation; spontaneous recovery in 40% of cases on catheter removal. Therapy only in symptomatic urinary tract infection in the presence of neu-

tropenia, after renal transplantation or before urologic surgery: fluconazole 200 mg/day for 14 days or amphotericin B 0.5 mg/kg/day for 7 days

- Candidaemia (clinically stable): remove or change CVC, fluconazole 400 mg/day i.v. for 7 days, then p.o. for at least 2 weeks after first negative blood culture; alternatively liposomal amphotericin B 3–5 mg/kg/day or voriconazole 400 mg p.o. q12h for 2 doses, then 200 mg
- Candidaemia (clinically unstable, treatment failure, above all *C. glabrata* or *C. krusei*, neutropenia): caspofungin 70 mg on day 1, 50 mg on day 2; anidulafungin 200 mg i.v. on day 1, then 100 mg/day i.v. or micafungin 100 mg/day i.v.; alternatively, fluconazole 800 mg (12 mg/kg) on day 1, then 400 mg (6 mg/kg) i.v.; voriconazole 6 mg/kg i.v. q12h on day 1, then 3 mg/kg i.v. q12h or amphotericin B 0.5–0.6 mg/kg/day i.v.
- Endocarditis, severe cases, metastases: liposomal amphotericin B 3–5 mg/kg/day i.v. ± flucytosine 25 mg/kg p.o. q6h; amphotericin B ± deoxycholate 0.6–1 mg/kg/day i.v. ± flucytosine 25 mg/kg p.o. q6h, caspofungin 70 mg on day 1, then 50 mg i.v. or anidulafungin 200 mg on day 1, then 100 mg/day or micafungin 100 mg/day

Remarks:

- NB antacids! With azole derivatives (exception: fluconazole) an acid gastric milieu is necessary for resorption
- Fluconazole is ineffective against *C. krusei* and only weakly active against *C. glabrata*
- Previous fluconazole therapy impairs the efficacy of amphotericin B against *C. albicans*
- Factors predisposing to candidiasis: diabetes mellitus, immune suppressive therapy, weakened autoimmunity (e.g. AIDS), wide-spectrum antibiotic therapy, long-term catheterisation; in urinary tract candidiasis always remove indwelling bladder catheter (blastomycetes are present in the catheter material and are inaccessible to antimycotic substances)
- Candidal endocarditis mostly arises in artificial heart valves; removal of the infected valve is almost always necessary

- In all systemic candidal infections, consider the possibility of metastatic–septic foci (endophthalmitis – ophthalmologic consultation)

Cat Scratch Fever

Most Frequent Pathogen:
Bartonella henselae

Primary Therapy:
Adults: 500 mg azithromycin q24h, then 250 mg/day for 4 days
Children: 10 mg/kg azithromycin q24h, then 5 mg/kg/day for 4 days

Remarks:
- No antibiotic therapy if course mild
- Complications: encephalitis, peripheral neuropathy, retinitis, endocarditis, granulomatous hepatitis, splenitis, interstitial pneumonia, osteitis

Cholangitis/Cholecystitis

Most Frequent Pathogens:
Enterobacteria, enterococci, *Clostridium* species, *Bacteroides*, *Ps. aeruginosa*

Primary Therapy:
Ampicillin/sulbactam, amoxicillin/clavulanic acid for 3–7 days

Alternatives:
Cephalosporins (3rd gen.) + metronidazole or clindamycin; piperacillin/tazobactam

Remarks:
Beware the biliary sludge phenomenon with ceftriaxone. Coverage for *Ps. aeruginosa* should be included in patients with

stents or history of endoscopy or surgical procedure. In life-threatening circumstances: preferably carbapenems.

Conjunctivitis (Purulent)

Most Frequent Pathogens:
Adults and children: *S. aureus*, pneumococci, *H. influenzae*, *Chlamydia trachomatis*, gonococci (very rarely)
Infants: staphylococci, *Ps. aeruginosa*, *Chlamydia trachomatis*, gonococci (very rarely)

Therapy:
- Adults and children:
  Quinolones (moxifloxacin, levofloxacin), locally
  Chlamydiae: doxycycline or erythromycin locally and p.o. for 1–3 weeks
  Gonococci: ceftriaxone 125 mg i.m. (single dose)
- Infants:
  Staphylococci: in light infections, local treatment (e.g. bacitracin ointment); in severe infections, flucloxacillin i.v. for 7–10 days
  Pseudomonas aeruginosa: in mild infections, local treatment (e.g. kanamycin eye drops); in severe infections, piperacillin, ceftazidime i.v. for 7–10 days
  Chlamydiae: erythromycin p.o. for 14 days (beware pneumonia!)
  Gonococci: local chloramphenicol eye ointment, simultaneously penicillin G or ceftriaxone i.v. for 7 days

Remarks:
- Gram staining and methylene blue staining usually provide important clues to the pathogen
- Three weeks after delivery gonococci are practically excluded. The cause of the conjunctivitis is then obstruction of the nasolacrimal duct by a staphylococcal superinfection (frequent)

- In contact lens wearers, especially those using the so-called "4-week lenses", conjunctivitis and keratitis are often caused by *Ps. aeruginosa*. Treatment: ciprofloxacin eye drops (every 15–60 min for 24–72 h)
- In case of chlamydiae and Gonococci, partner treatment is required

Cryptococcosis

Pathogen:
Cryptococcus neoformans

Primary Therapy:
Amphotericin B i.v. ± flucytosine p.o. for 6 weeks, then fluconazole for a further 8–10 weeks

Alternative:
In mild disease, fluconazole 400 mg/day i.v. or p.o. for at least 8 weeks

Remarks:
For prevention of recurrence in AIDS, fluconazole 200 mg/day for as long as required, if need be for life

Cystitis

▶ Urinary Tract Infections

Diabetic Foot

Most Frequent Pathogens:
Mixed aerobic–anaerobic infections, most frequently *S. aureus, Ps. aeruginosa, E. coli, B. fragilis*

Primary Therapy:
Local signs of infection: ampicillin/sulbactam + cotrimoxazole; or quinolone (group IV)
Local signs of infection + systemic involvement: carbapenem + vancomycin

Alternatives:
Local signs of infection: piperacillin/tazobactam (sulbactam) + cotrimoxazole; or quinolones (groups II, III) + clindamycin or Fosfomycin
Local signs of infection + systemic involvement: quinolone (groups III, IV) + vancomycin. If indicated, gram-positive coverage (including MRSA) can be achieved also with linezolid and daptomycin

Remarks:
- Exclude osteomyelitis
- Vascular surgery is usually necessary
- Sequential therapy is possible: 1–2 weeks i.v., then 3 weeks p.o.

Diphtheria

Pathogen:
Corynebacterium diphtheriae

Primary Therapy:
Penicillin G for 7–14 days + antitoxin

Alternative:
Erythromycin + antitoxin

Diverticulitis

Most Frequent Pathogens:
Enterobacteria, *Ps. aeruginosa*, *Bacteroides* species, enterococci

Primary Therapy:
a) Mild course, outpatient: amoxicillin/clavulanic acid p.o., or cotrimoxazole + metronidazole
b) Mild course, inpatient: ampicillin/sulbactam i.v.
c) Severe course: carbapenem or piperacillin/tazobactam

Alternatives:
a) Ciprofloxacin + metronidazole p.o.
b) Cephalosporin (2nd or 3rd gen.) + metronidazole i.v.; or ertapenem
c) Severe course: ampicillin + metronidazole + ciprofloxacin i.v.

Remarks:
- The pathogenetic significance of enterococci is controversial; substances effective against enterococci may be necessary only in patients at risk of endocarditis
- Exclude peritonitis
- Duration of therapy generally 7–10 days

Endocarditis

Most Frequent Pathogens:
- Adults:
  With pneumonia or meningitis: *S. aureus*, pneumococci, group A streptococci
  In i.v. drug abuse: *S. aureus, Ps. aeruginosa*, enterococci, *Candida albicans*
  Endocarditis in artificial heart valves:

- – <6 months after operation: S. *epidermidis, S. aureus,*
  diphtheroid bacteria, *Candida albicans*
- – >6 months after operation: viridans streptococci,
  enterococci, *S. aureus*, Gram-negative bacteria
- Children: viridans streptococci, enterococci, staphylococci,
  pneumococci, group A streptococci

Therapy:
▶ Chap. 11

Endometritis

Most Frequent Pathogens:
a) 1–48 h postpartum: amnionitis
b) 48 h to 6 weeks postpartum: *C. trachomatis, M. hominis*

Primary Therapy:
a) ▶ Amnionitis
b) Doxycycline 100 mg i.v. or p.o. q12h for 14 days

Remarks:
Discontinue breastfeeding if tetracyclines administered!

Endophthalmitis

Most Frequent Pathogens:
a) After surgery: *S. epidermidis* (60%), *S. aureus*, streptococci, *Ps. aeruginosa*; propionibacteria and coagulasen-
   egative staphylococci in chronic course
b) Endogenous (haematogenous): pneumococci, meningococci, *S. aureus*
c) Antibiotic therapy, indwelling catheter: *Candida species,*
   Aspergillus species

Primary Therapy:
a) Vancomycin + amikacin (intravitreal) or vancomycin + ceftazidime (intravitreal or, in severe cases, systemic)
b) Cephalosporin (3rd gen.) (systemic) + vancomycin (systemic and intravitreal)
c) Amphotericin B or voriconazole intravitreally, plus systemic therapy in moderate to severe infection

Remarks:
- Emergency: loss of sight possible within 24 h in severe cases
- Diabetes mellitus, chronic renal insufficiency, immune suppression, drug abuse: exclude fungal endophthalmitis
- Repeat intravitreal instillation a few days after vitrectomy
- Be aware of retinotoxiticy related to intravitreal application of amikacin
- Intravitreal dosages
  Amikacin 0.4 mg/0.1 ml;
  Ceftazidime 2 mg/0.1 ml;
  Vancomycin 1 mg/0.1 ml;
  Amphotericin B 5–7.5 µg/0.1 ml;
  Voriconazole 100 µg/0.1 ml

Enterocolitis (Pseudomembranous Clostridium difficile-associated Disease, CDAD)

Pathogen:
Clostridium difficile (particularly after antibiotic therapy)

Therapy:
If possible: discontinue the causative antibiotic, metronidazole 400 mg p.o. q8h, or metronidazole 250 mg i.v. q6h, or 500 mg i.v. q8h for 7–14 days
In severe cases (paralytic ileus): metronidazole 500 mg i.v. q6–8h + vancomycin 250–500 mg p.o. q6–8h

Alternative:
Vancomycin 125–250 mg p.o. q6–8h for 7–14 days

Remarks:
Because relapses are not related to development of resistance, another course of either oral metronidazole or vancomycin can be administered (same treatment for the same duration)

Epididymitis

Most Frequent Pathogens:
Age <35 years: gonococci, chlamydiae
Age >35 years: enterobacteria

Primary Therapy:
Age <35 years: 250 mg ceftriaxone i.m. as single dose + 100 mg doxycycline p.o. q12h for 10 days
Age >35 years: ciprofloxacin, ofloxacin, each for 10–14 days p.o. or i.v.

Alternatives:
Age <35 years: quinolones (groups I, II) p.o. for 10 days
Age >35 years: ampicillin/sulbactam, piperacillin/tazobactam, cephalosporins (3rd gen.)

Epiglottitis

Most Frequent Pathogens:
H. influenzae, S. pyogenes, pneumococci, *S. aureus*

Primary Therapy:
Cefuroxime, cefotaxime, ceftriaxone

Alternatives:
Ampicillin/sulbactam, cotrimoxazole

Remarks:
Most frequent pathogens in adults: group A streptococci; treatment as for children

Erysipelas

Most Frequent Pathogens:
Group A streptococci, rarely staphylococci

Primary Therapy:
Penicillin G 10–20 million IU/day i.v for severe cases; oral penicillins, 3 million IU/day for mild disease, for 10 days; benzathine penicillin once i.m., cephalosporins

Alternatives:
In penicillin allergy: macrolides; for staphylococcal infection: oxacillin, flucloxacillin

Remarks:
In case of frequent relapses, prophylaxis with benzathine penicillin once i.m., every 3–4 weeks is indicated

Gangrene

Pathogens:
Toxin-forming clostridia, particularly *C. perfringens*

Primary Therapy:
Penicillin G 24 million IU/day i.v. (in 4–6 doses) + clindamycin 900 mg i.v. q8h

Alternatives:
Ceftriaxone 2 g i.v. q12h, erythromycin 1 g i.v. q6h

Remarks:

Surgical consultation and intervention necessary. Clindamycin reduces toxin production. Hyperbaric oxygen therapy under discussion

Gastroenteritis

Most Frequent Pathogens:

- Blood, mucus and leukocytes in stool: *Campylobacter jejuni,* salmonellae, shigellae, amoebas, *Clostridium difficile,* EHEC (=enterohaemorrhagic *E. coli* O 157/H7; haemolytic–uraemic syndrome), *Yersinia enterocolitica*
- No leukocytes in stool: viruses (90% noroviruses, rarely rotaviruses in adults), rarely EPEC (enteropathogenic *E. coli*), vibrios, protozoa
- Travellers to Russia, America, Asia, Africa: *Campylobacter,* shigellae, salmonellae, *V. cholerae,* lambliae, *Cyclospora cayetanensis*

Primary Therapy:

- Adults:

  Salmonellae: generally no antibiotics; always replace water and electrolytes

  Shigellae: quinolones (after antibiogram)

  Campylobacter jejuni: in uncomplicated cases no antibiotics; otherwise erythromycin

  Yersinia enterocolitica: no antibiotics; in severe disease (bacteraemia) doxycycline, or cotrimoxazole or cephalosporins

  Amoebas: metronidazole + lumen-effective medication (► Amebiasis)

  Lambliae: metronidazole

  Vibrio cholerae: ciprofloxacin 1 g p.o. as single dose

  Cyclospora cayetanensis: cotrimoxazole

  Clostridium difficile (► Enterocolitis)

- Children:
  Salmonellae: no antibiotics
  Treatment only in infants, children with septic disease and patients with limited immune defences: cotrimoxazole or amoxicillin for 5–7 days
  EPEC: no chemotherapy, or colistin p.o. for 5–7 days
  EHEC: no antibiotics
  Campylobacter jejuni: in uncomplicated cases no antibiotics; otherwise erythromycin for 5–7 days
  Yersinia enterocolitica: no antibiotic therapy, or cotrimoxazole for 5–7 days
- Infants:
  EPEC: no antibiotics; if indicated: colistin, polymyxin B orally for 5 days
  EHEC: antibiotics contraindicated
  Salmonellae: ampicillin i.v. for 5–7 days
  Shigellae: ampicillin i.v. for 5–7 days (after antibiogram)

Alternatives:
- Adults:
  Shigellae: cotrimoxazole (after antibiogram), azithromycin
  Campylobacter jejuni: tetracyclines, azithromycin
  Yersinia enterocolitica: cotrimoxazole
- Children:
  Campylobacter jejuni: azithromycin, amoxicillin
  C. fetus: gentamicin, ceftriaxone, ampicillin

Remarks:
- Enteritis caused by salmonellae (e.g. *Salmonella enteritidis, S. typhimurium*): *do not treat with antibiotics!* Antibiotic therapy indicated only in infants, patients with massively compromised autoimmunity, and those over 70 years of age. In adults: 500 mg ciprofloxacin q12h, 500 mg levofloxacin p.o. q24h for 5 days (beware resistance). In asymptomatic salmonella excreters therapy can be tried in exceptional cases (e.g. food industry workers): ciprofloxacin 500 mg p.o. q12h for 5 days

- Antibiotic therapy in long-term excreters of *Salmonella typhi* and *Salmonella paratyphi* B: 3 months 2 tablets cotrimoxazole q12h or 2 weeks 750 mg ciprofloxacin q12h
- Traveller's diarrhoea: ciprofloxacin 750 mg or levofloxacin 500 mg or azithromycin 1 g as single dose (particularly for travellers in South-East Asia). In severe cases 500 mg ciprofloxacin p.o. q12h for 3 days; loperamide is contraindicated in mucohaemorrhagic diarrhoea
- Shigellae: NB: increasing resistance! Therefore, treatment after antibiogram if possible
- Do not treat uncomplicated *Campylobacter jejuni* infections (increasing resistance to quinolones and erythromycin)
- Never treat EHEC infections with antibiotics
- Amoebas amoebiasis (▶ Amebiasis)
- *Cyclospora cayetanensis*: cotrimoxazole forte 2 times daily for 7 days; in HIV, 4 times daily for 10 days

Gonorrhoea

Pathogen:
Neisseria gonorrheae

Therapy (uncomplicated cervicitis, urethritis, proctitis):
Ceftriaxone 125 mg i.m. q24h, cefotaxime 500 mg i.m. q24h, cefixime 400 mg p.o. q24h, ofloxacin 400 mg p.o. q24h, ciprofloxacin 500 mg p.o. q24h, levofloxacin 250 mg p.o. q24h (because of the frequent co-infection with *Chlamydia trachomatis*, it is recommended to add doxycycline 100 mg p.o. q12h for 7 days or azithromycin 1 g p.o. as a single dose)

Therapy (disseminated infection):
Ceftriaxone 2 g i.v. q24h or cefotaxime 1 g i.v. q8h or ciprofloxacin 400 mg i.v. q12h until 24 h after clinical improvement, then cefixime 400 mg p.o. q12h or ciprofloxacin 500 mg p.o. q12h for 7 days. Additional doxycycline or azithromycin for chlamydiae (above)

Remarks:
Gram staining and methylene blue staining often provide important clues to the pathogen. Treat the patient's sexual partner(s)!

Impetigo (Children, Infants)

Most Frequent Pathogens:
Group A streptococci, *S. aureus*

Primary Therapy:
No systemic antibiotics except in extended disease, in which case penicillin G (streptococci) or flucloxacillin (*S. aureus*) for 10 days, oral penicillins, oral cephalosporins (2nd gen.), macrolides

Remarks:
Local antibiotics: bacitracin or mupirocin ointment for 3–5 days

Keratitis

Most Frequent Pathogens:
a) Bacterial: *S. aureus*, *S. epidermidis*, *S. pneumoniae*, *S. pyogenes*, enterobacteria
b) Fungi: *Candida*, aspergilli, *Fusarium* species
c) Protozoa: *Acanthamoeba*
d) Contact lens wearers: *Ps. aeruginosa*

Primary Therapy:
a) Topical quinolones (e.g. moxifloxacin) or aminoglycosides (e.g. gentamicin)
b) Topical amphotericin B or natamycin
c) Topical aminoglycoside + propamidine isoethionate (Brolene®) or polyhexamethylene biguanide (PHMB, Lavasept®)
d) Topical aminoglycoside, piperacillin or ciprofloxacin

Remarks:
- Adenoviruses are the most frequent viral pathogens; differential diagnosis includes herpes simplex infection
- Application in bacterial keratitis: (incl. *Ps. aeruginosa*): every 15–60 min for 24–72 h, then gradual reduction
- Application in fungal keratitis: every 60 min with gradual reduction (extended treatment, possibly for months)
- Application in protozoal keratitis: every 30 min alternately for 72 h, then gradual reduction, treat for 1 year
- Systemic antibiotics only in severe disease with endophthalmitis

Lambliasis (Giardiasis)

Pathogen:
Giardia lamblia

Therapy:
Metronidazole 500 mg p.o. q8h for 5 days

Alternative:
Paromomycin 500 mg p.o. q6h for 7 days

Remarks:
Repeated treatment may be required; also treat asymptomatic excreters of cysts

Legionellosis

▶ Pneumonia

Leptospirosis

Pathogen:
Leptospira interrogans

Primary Therapy:
Penicillin G 1.5 million IU/day i.v. q6h for 7 days

Alternatives:
Ceftriaxone, doxycycline, ampicillin

Listeriosis

Pathogen:
Listeria monocytogenes

Primary Therapy:
Ampicillin 2–4 g i.v. q8h for 3–4 weeks + aminoglycoside in severe infection, especially in meningitis

Alternative:
Cotrimoxazole

Liver Abscess

Most Frequent Pathogens:
E. coli, *Proteus*, enterococci, *S. aureus*, *Bacteroides*, *Entamoeba histolytica*, *Streptococcus milleri*, echinococci

Primary Therapy:
Ampicillin + aminoglycosides + metronidazole

Alternatives:
Carbapenems, ampicillin/sulbactam, piperacillin/tazobactam or quinolones, each with metronidazole

Remarks:
Surgical consultation and possibly intervention necessary. Include serology for amoebas and echinococci in the diagnostic algorithm (▶ Amebiasis). If serology positive for amoebas, monotherapy with metronidazole (no surgery)

Lung Abscess

▶ Pneumonia

Mastitis

Most Frequent Pathogen:
S. aureus

Primary Therapy:
- Adults: cephalosporins, flucloxacillin for 1 week
- Infants: dicloxacillin, flucloxacillin, older 2nd generation cephalosporins for 1 week

Alternatives:
- Adults: clindamycin

Remarks:
Surgical consultation and possibly intervention necessary. Gram staining and methylene blue staining usually provide important clues to the pathogen
Infants: Gram staining of colostrums, incision often necessary
Mastitis at times other than lactation: clindamycin is first choice, as the pathogen may be *Bacteroides*
Mastitis without abscess: not necessary to discontinue breast-feeding

Mastoiditis

Most Frequent Pathogen:
Acute: pneumococci, *S. aureus*, *H. influenzae*, group A streptococci, *Ps. aeruginosa*
Chronic: anaerobes, *Ps. aeruginosa*, enterobacteria, *S. aureus*, often polymicrobial!

Primary Therapy:
Acute: surgery indicated; accompanying antibiotic therapy as for acute otitis media; in severe cases cephalosporins (3rd gen.)
Chronic: surgery indicated; accompanying antibiotic therapy with piperacillin/tazobactam or carbapenems

Remarks:
ENT consultation indispensable

Meningitis

Most Frequent Pathogens:
a) Adults <50 years of age and children >1 month: pneumococci, meningococci, *H. influenzae*
b) Neonates: (<1 month): group B streptococci, *E. coli*, listeriae, Gram-negative and Gram-positive pathogens
c) Adults >50 years of age: diabetes, alcoholism, immune suppression, pregnancy: pneumococci, listeriae, Gram-negative pathogens
d) After neurosurgery or trauma: pneumococci, *S. aureus*, *Ps. aeruginosa*, Gram-negative bacteria
e) Ventriculitis/meningitis owing to infected ventriculoparietal shunt: *S. epidermidis*, *S. aureus*, Gram-negative bacteria, *Propionibacterium acnes*

Primary Therapy:
a) Ceftriaxone (adults: 2 g q12h; children: 50 mg/kg q12h) or cefotaxime (adults: 3–4 g q8h; children: 200 mg/kg/day) + ampicillin (until listeriae excluded)
b) Ampicillin (50 mg/kg q6–8h) + cefotaxime (50 mg/kg q6–8h)
c) Ampicillin (4 g q8h) + ceftriaxone (2 g q12h)
d) Vancomycin (adults: 500 mg q6h; children: 15 mg/kg q6h) + ceftazidime (adults: 2 g q8h; children: 50 mg/kg q8h)
e) Children: vancomycin (15 mg/kg q6h) + ceftriaxone (50 mg/kg q12h)

Adults: vancomycin (1 g q6–12h) + rifampin (600 mg/day p.o.); remove shunt!

Alternatives:

a) Meropenem (adults: 2 g q8h; children: 40 mg/kg q8h). NB: occasional convulsions!
b) Ampicillin (50 mg/kg q6–8h) + gentamicin (2.5 mg/kg q12–24h)
c) Meropenem (2 g q8h; NB: occasional convulsions!)
d) Meropenem (2 g q8h; NB: occasional convulsions!) + vancomycin (1 g q12h)
e) Meropenem (2 g q8h; NB: occasional convulsions!) + vancomycin (1 g q12h)
   Duration of treatment: 7–10 days; in postoperative meningitis at least 10 days; in listerial meningitis 21 days

Remarks:

- Always obtain blood for culture. Gram staining and methylene blue staining usually provide important clues to the pathogen. Current pneumococcal resistance Chap. 7
- Meningitis prophylaxis p. 282
- Penicillin allergy: chloramphenicol (if meningococci suspected) + cotrimoxazole (if listeriae suspected) + vancomycin
- Administration of dexamethasone, particularly in *H. influenzae* meningitis, reduces late neurologic sequelae in infants, especially hearing loss. Recommended for adult patients in pneumococcal and meningococcal meningitis. Dosage for all age groups: 0.15 mg/kg i.v. q6h for 4 days, always 15–20 min before antibiotic administration
- In postoperative meningitis with coliform bacteria or *Ps. aeruginosa* it may be appropriate to give gentamicin 4 mg q12h each day intrathecally until the CSF is sterile
- When pathogen is known:
  Pneumococci: penicillin (penicillin allergy: vancomycin + rifampin), ceftriaxone or cefotaxime.
  In case of penicillin-resistant pneumococci with MIC ≥2 mcq/ml add vancomycin to ceftriaxone
  Meningococci: penicillin

H. influenzae: ampicillin
Listeriae: ampicillin + aminoglycosides
Ps. aeruginosa: ceftazidime + aminoglycosides
Group B streptococci: penicillin ± aminoglycosides
S. aureus: flucloxacillin ± rifampin or fosfomycin
S. epidermidis: vancomycin, teicoplanin, flucloxacillin (antibiogram!)
C. albicans: liposomal amphotericin B (3–5 mg/kg) ± flucytosine (25 mg/kg) followed by fluconazole 400–800 mg

10

Necrotising Fasciitis, Toxic Shock Syndrome

Pathogens:
a) *S. aureus* (staphylococcal toxic shock syndrome)
b) Streptococci of groups A, B, C, G (streptococcal toxic shock syndrome)
c) Aerobic–anaerobic mixed infections (necrotising fasciitis)
d) Clostridia

Therapy:
a) Flucloxacillin 12 g/day i.v.
b) Penicillin G 24 million IU/day i.v. + clindamycin 900 mg i.v. q8h + immunoglobulins or ceftriaxone 2 g/day i.v. + clindamycin i.v. + immunoglobulins
c) Meropenem, imipenem
d) Penicillin G 24 million IU/day i.v. + clindamycin 900 mg i.v. q8h

Remarks:
Mortality in fasciitis 30–50%, in myositis 80%; clindamycin inhibits the toxin production of streptococci, surgical intervention (debridement, excision, filleting incisions, amputation) In countries with high prevalence of MRSA in the community, consider empiric therapy with glycopeptides, linezolid or daptomycin

Nocardiosis

Pathogens:
Nocardia species
Therapy:
- Cutaneous nocardiosis:
  Cotrimoxazole (5–10 mg/kg/day TMP + 25–50 mg/kg/day SMX) i.v. or p.o. in 2–4 doses
  or
  minocycline 100–200 mg p.o. q12h
- Pulmonary, systemic, cerebral nocardiosis:
  Cotrimoxazole (initially 15 mg/kg/day TMP + 75 mg/kg/day SMX for 3–4 weeks, then 10 mg/kg/day TMP + 50 mg/kg/day SMX) i.v. or p.o. in 2–4 doses ± ceftriaxone 2 g q12h
  or
  Imipenem 500 mg i.v. q6h + amikacin 7.5 mg/kg q12h for 3–4 weeks, then continue with cotrimoxazole or minocycline p.o.

Remarks:
- Consider nocardiae particularly in patients with weakened autoimmunity (e.g. cytostatic therapy) and lung findings
- Duration of treatment in immunocompetent patients 3 months, in immune-suppressed patients 6 months; possible alternative: 600 mg linezolid q12h
- Endocarditis: imipenem + amikacin for 2 months, then cotrimoxazole for 4 months (single case report)

Orbital Phlegmon

Most Frequent Pathogens:
S. aureus, group A streptococci, *H. influenzae* (children <5 years of age), pneumococci, *M. catarrhalis*, anaerobes, Gram-negative bacteria (following trauma)

Primary Therapy:
Cephalosporins (2nd/3rd gen.) + metronidazole, ampicillin/sulbactam

---

Osteomyelitis

1. Acute Osteomyelitis

Most Frequent Pathogens:
a) Adults: *S. aureus*
b) Children >4 months: *S. aureus*, group A streptococci, rarely Gram-negative bacteria
c) Children <4 months: *S. aureus*, Gram-negative bacteria, group B streptococci
d) Adults with sickle cell anaemia/thalassaemia: *Salmonella* species
e) Patients with haemodialysis, drug addiction, diabetes mellitus: *S. aureus*, *Ps. aeruginosa*
f) After trauma, in soft tissue infection: polymicrobial (incl. anaerobes)
g) After surgical treatment of a fracture: Gram-negative bacteria, *S. aureus*, *Ps. aeruginosa*
h) After sternotomy: *S. aureus*, *S. epidermidis*

Primary Therapy:
a) Flucloxacillin/oxacillin/cefazolin (MSSA), glycopeptides (MRSA)
b) Flucloxacillin + cephalosporin (3rd gen.), glycopeptides (MRSA)
c) Flucloxacillin + cephalosporin (3rd gen.), glycopeptides (MRSA)
d) Quinolones
e) Flucloxacillin/oxacillin + ciprofloxacin, glycopeptides (MRSA)
f) Ampicillin/sulbactam, amoxicillin/clavulanic acid, piperacillin/tazobactam or piperacillin/sulbactam or cephalosporins + metronidazole, glycopeptides (MRSA)

g) Flucloxacillin/oxacillin + ciprofloxacin, glycopeptides (MRSA)
h) Vancomycin or teicoplanin + rifampin

Alternatives:
a) Cephalosporin (2nd gen.), quinolones + rifampin (MSSA)
b) Clindamycin ± cephalosporin (3rd gen.), quinolones + rifampin (MSSA)
c) Clindamycin + cephalosporin (3rd gen.), quinolones + rifampin (MSSA)
d) Cephalosporins (3rd gen.)
e) Vancomycin + ciprofloxacin, quinolones + rifampin (MSSA), piperacillin/tazobactam (*Pseudomonas*)
f) Carbapenem
g) Vancomycin + cephalosporin (3rd gen.) effective against *Pseudomonas* or piperacillin/tazobactam
h) Linezolid

Remarks:
- Microbiological cultures are essential
- High MRSA rate vancomycin or teicoplanin. Some data support use of linezolid and daptomycin for osteomyelitis due to MRSA
- Surgical debridement is practically always necessary (exception: haematogenous osteomyelitis in children)
- Duration of treatment: 6–8 weeks (in children with haematogenous osteomyelitis 3 weeks' therapy generally suffices, the first 2 weeks i.v.)
- Switch from i.v. to oral administration after subsidence of fever, disappearance of pain, and normalisation of leukocyte count, left displacement and CRP value
- No switch to oral therapy in patients with diabetes or severe peripheral vascular disease
- In culture-negative osteomyelitis, especially in children, consider *Kingella kingae*
- If therapy fails, always exclude tuberculosis
- Neonates with osteomyelitis are often afebrile (risk factors: artificial respiration, premature birth)

- So-called small colony variants (SCV) of *S. aureus* display distinctly retarded growth on conventional culture media. They are characterised by reduced antibiotic sensitivity and a high potential for recurring infection (which may be induced by use of gentamicin-impregnated PMMA)

2. Chronic Osteomyelitis

Most Frequent Pathogens:
S. aureus, enterobacteria, *Ps. aeruginosa*

Remarks:
- Treatment for up to 6 months may be necessary
- Always specific therapy after identification of pathogen
- Debridement

3. Osteomyelitis after Joint Implantation

Most Frequent Pathogens:
Streptococci, *S. aureus*, *S. epidermis*, *Ps. aeruginosa*

Empirical Therapy:
Treatment according to microbiological findings

Specific Therapy (always aim to identify pathogen):
- MSSA: oxacillin or flucloxacillin i.v. + rifampin i.v. for 2–4 weeks, then ciprofloxacin or levofloxacin p.o. + rifampin p.o.
- MRSA: vancomycin i.v. + rifampin p.o. for 2–4 weeks, then cotrimoxazole (or fusidic acid or ciprofloxacin or levofloxacin) p.o. + rifampin p.o.
- Streptococci: penicillin G i.v. or ceftriaxone for 4 weeks, then amoxicillin p.o.
- Anaerobes: clindamycin i.v. for 2–4 weeks, then clindamycin p.o.
- *Ps. aeruginosa*: ceftazidime i.v. ± aminoglycosides i.v. for 2–4 weeks, then ciprofloxacin p.o.
- Other Gram-negative pathogens: ciprofloxacin p.o.
- Mixed flora: imipenem or piperacillin/tazobactam for 2–4 weeks, then p.o. according to the antibiogram

Remarks:
- In chronic/insidious implant infection there is generally no leukocytosis and no left displacement
- Intraoperative culture of biopsy samples only on suspicion of infection
- An infection can be diagnosed only after several positive biopsies and/or histological demonstration of purulent inflammation
- Surgical intervention is necessary if antibiotic therapy is to be successful. With early infection and a stable prosthesis, debridement combined with antibiotic treatment suffices; otherwise the infected implant must be replaced. With low-virulent pathogens and favourable bone and tissue conditions, exchange in a single session can be attempted.
- Duration of treatment: at least 3 months in internal fixations and hip joint prostheses, at least 6 months in knee implants; always continue antibiotic therapy for at least 1 month after normalisation of leukocyte count, CRP value and clinical signs of infection

Otitis Externa

Most Frequent Pathogens:
Ps. aeruginosa, *Proteus*, streptococci, staphylococci

Primary Therapy:
In mild forms of otitis externa ("swimmer's ear"), local application of, for example, Dexa-Polyspectran in the cleansed external meatus. If symptoms worsen, use ciprofloxacin ear drops; hydrocortisone

Remarks:
Always consult an ENT specialist. If primary therapy fails: *Pseudomonas*-active penicillins (e.g. piperacillin) or cephalosporins (e.g. ceftazidime)
NB Otitis externa maligna (e.g. in diabetics): always use antibiotics active against *Pseudomonas* in combination with aminoglycosides

Otitis Media

Most Frequent Pathogens:
- Adults and children: viruses (up to 50%), pneumococci, *H. influenzae* (more frequent in children), streptococci, moraxellae
- Infants: Gram-negative bacteria, staphylococci, *H. influenzae*, streptococci, pneumococci

Primary Therapy (in bacterial infection):
Ampicillin/sulbactam, amoxicillin/clavulanic acid

Alternatives:
- Adults and children: oral cephalosporins (2nd gen.); azithromycin (children: 30 mg/kg as single dose); ceftriaxone

Remarks:
- Children should primarily receive analgesics rather than antibiotics. Give antibiotics only if there is no improvement by the next day (6 months to 2 years of age) or by the 3rd day (>2 years of age). This does not apply to children with poor general condition or otorrhea (NB: mastoiditis!)
- Duration of therapy: children <2 years of age: 10 days; children ≥2 years of age: 5–7 days; shorter courses with azithromycin (3–5 days) or ceftriaxone i.m. for 3 days; ceftriaxone 50 mg/kg i.m. as a single dose proven only for children aged 7–21 months
- Penicillin-resistant pneumococci: increase amoxicillin dosage to 80 mg/kg/day in 3 doses. Current pneumococcal resistance ▶ Chap. 7

Pancreatitis (Acute, Chronic)

Most Frequent Pathogens:
Mostly not bacterial in origin (alcohol!); enterobacteria, enterococci, *S. aureus*, *S. epidermidis*, anaerobes, *Candida* species

Primary Therapy:
Alcoholic aetiology, no necroses: no antibiotic therapy
Necroses and infected pseudocysts, or infected necroses:
carbapenems for 2(–4) weeks

Alternatives:
Quinolones (groups II, III) + metronidazole, cephalosporins +
metronidazole

Remarks:
Surgical consultation and possibly intervention necessary

Parotitis (Bacterial)

Most Frequent Pathogens:
S. aureus, streptococci, *H. influenzae*, oral flora

Therapy:
Cephalosporin (2nd gen.), oxacillin, amoxicillin/clavulanic acid,
ampicillin/sulbactam for 14 days

Remarks:
Differential diagnosis: granulomatous inflammation (atypical
mycobacteria, fungi, sarcoidosis, Sjögren syndrome, tumour):
no signs of inflammation, treatment after histology

Pericarditis

Most Frequent Pathogens:
- Adults: viruses, *S. aureus*, pneumococci, group A streptococci, Gram-negative bacteria, tubercle bacilli, rickettsiae,
  chlamydiae, *Coxiella burnetii*, mycoplasmas
- Children: staphylococci, *H. influenzae*, pneumococci, meningococci, streptococci, Gram-negative bacteria

Therapy (Purulent Pericarditis):
Primary therapy
Oxacillin (or flucloxacillin) + ciprofloxacin for 4–6 weeks

Alternatives
Vancomycin + ciprofloxacin for 4–6 weeks (high risk of MRSA); with tubercle bacilli, ▶ Tuberculosis

Remarks:
Surgical consultation and possibly intervention necessary. Gram stain or methylene blue stain mostly gives important clues to the pathogen. Order numerous cultures (anaerobes, fungi, TB) and serologic investigations (rickettsiae, ornithoses, syphilis, viruses)

Peritonitis

Most Frequent Pathogens:
a) Primary, spontaneously bacterial: enterobacteria (60%), pneumococci (15%), enterococci (10%), anaerobes (<1%)
b) Secondary: enterobacteria, enterococci, *Bacteroides*
c) In CAPD: most frequently *S. aureus*, *S. epidermidis*, *Ps. aeruginosa*, Gram-negative pathogens

Primary Therapy:
a) Ampicillin/sulbactam, piperacillin/tazobactam or piperacillin/sulbactam for 5–14 days
b) Cephalosporins (2nd/3rd gen.) + metronidazole, ertapenem for 5–7 days
c) Cephalosporins (3rd gen.) + vancomycin (intraperitoneally, in severe cases + i.v.)

Alternatives:
a) Cefotaxime, ceftriaxone
b) Ampicillin/sulbactam, piperacillin/tazobactam, carbapenems, quinolones + metronidazole, quinolones (group IV)
c) Vancomycin + aminoglycoside

Remarks:
Around 30% of patients with liver cirrhosis and ascites suffer primary peritonitis (give antibiotics at >250 cells/mm^3) within a year. Occasionally fungi can also cause primary peritonitis. At a high rate of ESBL-positive Klebsiellae and *E. coli*, give carbapenems. Surgical consultation and possibly intervention necessary. Gram staining or methylene blue staining mostly gives important clues to the pathogen. Blood cultures are useful in determining pathogen aetiology. Prophylaxis of spontaneously bacterial peritonitis, p. 282

Pertussis

Pathogen:
Bordetella pertussis

Primary Therapy:
Children: erythromycin estolate 40 mg/kg/day in 3 doses for 14 days
Adults: azithromycin 500 mg on day 1, 250 mg on days 2–5

Alternatives:
Cotrimoxazole (in erythromycin intolerance) for 14 days; clarithromycin for 7 days

Remarks:
Of adults with cough persisting >14 days, 10–15% have pertussis

Pleural Empyema

Most Frequent Pathogens:
Pneumococci, group A streptococci, *S. aureus*, enterobacteria, anaerobes (in chronic empyema)

Primary Therapy:
Cephalosporins (3rd gen.) ± clindamycin

Alternatives:
Amoxicillin/clavulanic acid, ampicillin/sulbactam, piperacillin/tazobactam, vancomycin, carbapenems

Remarks:
Surgical consultation and possibly intervention (chest tube drainage) necessary. Gram staining or methylene blue staining mostly gives important clues to the pathogen. Current pneumococcal resistance ▶ Chap. 7

Pneumonia

Most Frequent Pathogens:
- Adults:
  a) Community-acquired, no risk factors: pneumococci, mycoplasmas, chlamydiae, *H. influenzae*, moraxellae, legionellae, viruses
  b) Community-acquired, risk factors (age >60, diabetes, alcoholism) present: pneumococci, *H. influenzae*, mycoplasmas, legionellae, chlamydiae, moraxellae, polymicrobial; aspiration risk!
  c) Nosocomial: without artificial respiration: pneumococci, *H. influenzae*, *K. pneumoniae*, *S. aureus*. With artificial respiration: *Ps. aeruginosa*, *S. aureus*, *Enterobacter* species, *Acinetobacter* species, klebsiellae, *Candida albicans* (especially in neutropenia and with antibiotic therapy >1 week), legionellae
  d) Aspiration pneumonia with or without abscess: *Bacteroides* species, peptostreptococci, *Fusobacterium* species, *Streptococcus milleri* group
- Children:
  a) Age 1–3 months: *C. trachomatis*, viruses
  b) Age 4 months to 5 years: viruses, pneumococci, *H. influenzae*, mycoplasmas, chlamydiae

   c) Age 5–18 years: mycoplasmas, pneumococci, chlamydiae

Primary Therapy:
- Adults:
  - a) Amoxicillin-clavulanate, macrolides
  - b) Cephalosporins (3rd gen.) + macrolide or levofloxacin
  - c) Without artificial respiration: cephalosporins (2nd/3rd gen.) ± vancomycin (high suspicion of MRSA).
    With artificial respiration: ceftazidime ± aminoglycoside or in combination with quinolone ± vancomycin (high suspicion of MRSA).
  - d) Cephalosporins (2nd gen.) + metronidazole
- Children:
  - a) Macrolides (+ cefotaxime in high fever) for 10–14 days
  - b) (Oral) cephalosporin (2nd gen.) + macrolide or ciprofloxacin (not approved)
  - c) Macrolides [if pneumococci suspected, + (oral) cephalosporin]

Alternatives:
- Adults:
  - a) Ampicillin/sulbactam + macrolide, quinolones (group III or IV)
  - b) Piperacillin/tazobactam or carbapenems in combination with macrolide, quinolones (group III or IV)
  - c) Without artificial respiration: quinolones (group III or IV) or ampicillin-sulbactam ± linezolid (high suspicion of MRSA)
    With artificial respiration: piperacillin/tazobactam or cefepime or carbapenems in combination with aminoglycoside or ciprofloxacin ± linezolid (high suspicion of MRSA)
  - d) Ampicillin/sulbactam, carbapenems, quinolones (group IV), piperacillin/tazobactam

Remarks:

- Current pneumococcal resistance ▶ Chap. 7. In (partial) penicillin resistance: cefotaxime, ceftriaxone, cefepime, or quinolones (group III or IV)
- Blood cultures often indicate aetiology of pathogen; however the usefulness of blood culture in uncomplicated community-acquired pneumonia is controversial
- Purulent excretion: suspicion of lung abscess with anaerobes
- Mycoplasmas are relatively frequent in young adults and children >5 years of age; therefore give macrolides empirically
- In immunocompromised patients, *Pneumocystis jiroveci*: Mycobacteria and fungi need to be included in the diagnostic algorithm
- *Pneumocystis jiroveci* (*carinii*) pneumonia: 15–20 mg/kg/day trimethoprim + 75–100 mg/kg/day sulfamethoxazole in 3–4 doses for 21 days (first 48 h i.v.) + folic acid ± prednisolone Alternative: pentamidine 4 mg/kg/day i.v. for 21 days
- *Legionella* pneumonia: azithromycin 500 mg p.o. q24h for at least 5 days. In severe pneumonia: erythromycin 0.5–1 g q6h ± rifampin 600 mg/day for 14 days or clarithromycin 500 mg q12h for 14 days or levofloxacin 500 mg i.v. q12h for 7–14 days or ciprofloxacin 400 mg q8h for 10 days
- Psittacosis (*Chlamydia psittaci*): doxycycline or macrolides for 2 weeks
- *Candida* pneumonia: ▶ Candidiasis
- Infants: in interstitial pneumonia, cytomegalovirus is not infrequently accompanied by *Pneumocystis jiroveci* (*carinii*) (trimethoprim 20 mg/kg/day and sulfamethoxazole 100 mg/kg/day or pentamidine 4 mg/kg/day)

Prostatitis

Most Frequent Pathogens:
Acute: enterobacteria, *C. trachomatis, N. gonorrhoeae*
Chronic: enterobacteria, enterococci, *Ps. aeruginosa*

Primary Therapy:
Acute: quinolones p.o. for 10–14 days
Chronic: quinolones p.o. for 4 weeks, e.g. ciprofloxacin 500 mg p.o. q12h, norfloxacin 400 mg p.o. q12h, levofloxacin 500 mg p.o. q24h

Alternatives:
Acute: cotrimoxazole 1DS (TMP160mg) p.o. q12h for 10–14 days
Chronic: cotrimoxazole1DS (TMP160mg) q12h for (1–)3 months

Remarks:
Gonococci and chlamydiae are frequent in men <35 years of age (therapy ▶ Gonorrhoea)

Pyelonephritis

Most Frequent Pathogens:
Acute: *E. coli* (80%), other enterobacteria
Chronic, recurring: *E. coli*, *Proteus*, *Klebsiella*, enterococci

Primary Therapy:

Acute: Mild: quinolones p.o. for 7 days;
          Severe: cephalosporins (3rd gen.) i.v. for 10–14 days or quinolones i.v. for 10–14 days

Chronic, recurring: oral cephalosporins for 4–6 weeks

Alternatives:

Acute: Mild: oral cephalosporins for 7 days;
          Severe: piperacillin/tazobactam for 10–14 days

Chronic, recurring: amoxicillin/clavulanic acid, ampicillin/sulbactam, quinolones for 4–6 weeks

Remarks:

- Cephalosporins are ineffective against enterococci, so microbiological diagnosis is necessary
- Acute: microscopic and bacteriologic examination of urine 3–5 days after start of therapy (by which time urine should be sterile); i.v. therapy until 1–2 days after subsidence of fever, then switch to oral administration
- Chronic: microscopic and bacteriologic examination of urine weekly until 3 weeks after the end of therapy, then monthly for 3 months, then three times at 6-month intervals
- In chronic recurring urinary tract infection (e.g., recurrence only 1–3 weeks after discontinuation of chemotherapy), exclude obstruction and take measures to prevent reinfection: after elimination of the pathogen, give the antibiotic at one third of the usual daily dose (e.g. 50–100 mg nitrofurantoin or 1 tablet cotrimoxazole) without interruption (for at least 6 months), to be taken once daily after the evening meal

Q Fever

Pathogen:
Coxiella burnetii

Therapy:
Acute: doxycycline 100 mg p.o. q12h or i.v. for 14–21 days; quinolones in meningoencephalitis
Endocarditis or chronic form: doxycycline + chloroquine for at least 18 months

Remarks:
In acute hepatitis accompanying Q fever, administration of prednisone 40 mg/day for 7 days is advisable because of the strong immune response; in chronic Q fever, monitor antibodies every 3 months

Salpingitis (Adnexitis, Pelvic Inflammatory Disease)

Most Frequent Pathogens:
Gonococci, chlamydiae, *Bacteroides* species, enterobacteria, streptococci, mycoplasmas

Primary Therapy (outpatient):
Ceftriaxone 250 mg i.m. or i.v. as single dose, then doxycycline p.o. ± metronidazole

Primary Therapy (inpatient):
Cephalosporin (2nd gen.) i.v. + doxycycline p.o. for 10–14 days

Alternatives (outpatient):
Quinolone (group II, III) + metronidazole

Alternatives (inpatient):
Ampicillin/sulbactam i.v. or ertapenem i.v. + doxycycline p.o.; clindamycin + gentamicin, then doxycycline

Remarks:
- Duration of therapy: 10–14 days
- Possibly treat partner
- In pregnancy: macrolides instead of doxycyline
- Laparoscopy if noninvasive diagnosis is inconclusive

Scarlet Fever

▶ Tonsillitis

Sepsis

Most Frequent Pathogens:
- Adults:
  a) Venous catheter sepsis: *S. aureus, S. epidermidis, Candida albicans* (particularly in hyperalimentation)
  b) Urosepsis: enterobacteria (mostly *E. coli*), enterococci; after urologic surgery: *Proteus, Serratia, Enterobacter, Ps. aeruginosa*
  c) Wound infection sepsis: staphylococci, streptococci, *E. coli*; anaerobes
  d) In neutropenia: *S. epidermidis*, enterobacteria, *Ps. aeruginosa, Candida albicans*
  e) Pulmonary sepsis: pneumococci, *S. aureus*, klebsiellae; in artificial respiration: *Ps. aeruginosa, S. aureus*
  f) Puerperal sepsis (septic abortion): mixed aerobic–anaerobic infection, chlamydiae
  g) Abdominal sepsis: enterobacteria, anaerobes, enterococci; after ERCP, often *Ps. aeruginosa*
- Infants and children:
  Staphylococci, streptococci, pneumococci, meningococci, *H. influenzae, E. coli, Ps. aeruginosa, Klebsiella pneumoniae, Candida* species
- Neonates:
  Age <1 week: group B-streptococci, *E. coli, Klebsiella* species, *Enterobacter* species,
  Age 1–4 weeks: as above, but also *H. influenzae, S. epidermidis*

Primary Therapy:
- Adults:
  SIRS, unidentified focus: imipenem or meropenem (± vancomycin)
  a) Vancomycin (*Candida* sepsis, ▶ Candidiasis)
  b) Cephalosporin (3rd gen.), piperacillin/tazobactam, ampicillin/sulbactam

  c) Cephalosporin (2nd gen.), ampicillin/sulbactam ± metronidazole
  d) Pseudomonas-active cephalosporin (e.g. ceftazidime) or penicillin (e.g. piperacillin) ± vancomycin or teicoplanin (high risk MRSA) ± aminoglycoside
  e) Cephalosporin (2nd/3rd gen.) (± aminoglycoside) + macrolide if community acquired
  f) Ampicillin/sulbactam + doxycycline
  g) Cephalosporin (3rd gen.) + metronidazole, piperacillin/tazobactam

Continue treatment in all cases until 3–5 days (neutropenia: 7 days) after fever subsides; for *S. aureus*: 4 weeks

- Infants and children:
  Cephalosporin (3rd gen.)
- Neonates:
  Ampicillin + ceftriaxone

Alternatives:

Unidentified focus: piperacillin/tazobactam or piperacillin/sulbactam ± aminoglycoside or ± daptomycin, cephalosporin (3rd gen.) ± aminoglycoside

- Adults:
  a) Daptomycin, quinupristin/dalfopristin
  b) Quinolones (group II/III), carbapenems
  c) Ampicillin/sulbactam, piperacillin/tazobactam or piperacillin/sulbactam, carbapenems (sepsis secondary to abdominal surgery)
  d) Meropenem, imipenem ± aminoglycoside ± vancomycin
  e) Ampicillin/sulbactam, piperacillin/tazobactam, each ± aminoglycoside ± vancomycin or linezolid (high risk of MRSA)
  f) Cephalosporins (3rd gen.) + clindamycin, ertapenem + doxycycline
  g) Quinolones (group II/III) + metronidazole, imipenem, meropenem
- Infants and children:
  Flucloxacillin + cefuroxime

- Neonates:
  Ampicillin + cefotaxime

Remarks:
- Combination therapy with aminoglycosides whenever condition is life-threatening and/or a Gram-negative pathogen is probable, and always in presence of *Ps. aeruginosa*, *Acinetobacter* and *Serratia*
- Venous catheterisation, artificial respiration and bladder catheterisation are the most frequent causes of nosocomial sepsis; therefore remove catheter if at all possible if link to sepsis seems likely
- Nontunnelled/nonimplanted venous catheters: try catheter lock therapy (below) only with *S. epidermidis*; otherwise, remove catheter
- Tunnelled/implanted venous catheters: try catheter lock therapy (below) only in uncomplicated infections; otherwise, remove catheter
- Fungal sepsis: always remove catheter (▶ Candidiasis)
- Catheter lock therapy (only in combination with antibiotic therapy!): 50–100 IU heparin in 5 ml NaCl + vancomycin (1–5 mg/ml) or + gentamicin (1–2 mg/ml) or + ciprofloxacin (1–2 mg/ml). Fill the catheter lumen (2–5 ml) with this solution between antibiotic doses or, for example, 12 h overnight; remove solution from catheter before giving medication; duration of therapy: 2 weeks
- Methicillin-susceptible *S. aureus* sepsis: vancomycin is less effective than oxacillin or flucloxacillin; beware endocarditis, particularly with CVC
- Septic shock in parenteral nutrition: always check for contamination of infusion! Send remaining infusion fluid for bacteriologic examination
- In neutropenic patients with fever after 5 days of empiric antibiotic therapy consider to add antifungal therapy (▶ Candidiasis).
- In infants always exclude accompanying meningitis or UTI

Sinusitis

Most Frequent Pathogens:
Acute: pneumococci, *H. influenzae*, moraxellae, staphylococci
Chronic: Staphylococci, streptococci, *H. influenzae*, anaerobes

Primary Therapy:
Acute: amoxicillin ± clavulanic acid, ampicillin ± sulbactam for 10–14 days
Chronic: antibiotic therapy frequently ineffective; acute exacerbations: as for acute disease

Alternatives:
Acute: Oral cephalosporins (2nd/3rd gen.), clindamycin, quinolones (group III, IV)

Syphilis

Pathogen:
Treponema pallidum

Primary Therapy:
Early syphilis (<1 year):
Benzathine penicillin: 2.4 million IU i.m. as single dose
Penicillin allergy:
- Doxycycline 100 mg p.o. q12h or tetracyclines 500 mg q6h for 14 days
- Ceftriaxone 1 g/day i.m. or i.v. for 8–10 days

Late syphilis (>1 year):
Benzathine penicillin G: 2.4 million IU i.m. weekly for 3 weeks
Penicillin allergy:
- Doxycycline 100 mg p.o. q12h for 28 days
- Tetracyclines 500 mg p.o. q6h for 28 days

Syphilis in pregnancy:
Benzathine penicillin G: 2.4 million IU i.m.
Penicillin allergy:
- Ceftriaxone 250 mg/day i.m. for 10 days (exclude parallel allergies!)

Neurosyphilis:
Penicillin G: 5 million IU/day i.v. q6h for 10–14 days

Congenital syphilis:
Penicillin G: 100,000–150,000 IU/kg/day i.v. in 2–3 doses or procaine penicillin G: 50,000 IU/kg/day i.m., each for at least 10–14 days

Remarks:
In infants always obtain a sample of CSF to exclude CNS involvement

---

Tetanus

Pathogen:
Clostridium tetani

Primary Therapy:
Metronidazole 500 mg/day q6h for 7–10 days + antitoxin 6,000 IU i.m. + immunoglobulin

Alternatives:
Penicillin G 24 million IU/day for 10 days, tetracyclines

Remarks:
Muscle relaxation with diazepam. Postexposure prophylaxis
▶ p. 286

Tonsillitis, Purulent

Most Frequent Pathogens:
Group A streptococci

Primary Therapy:
Penicillin V for 10 days

Alternatives:
Oral cephalosporins (2nd gen.) or macrolides

Remarks:
Resistance of streptococci to macrolides is on the increase in Europe
Repeated detection of group A streptococci in tonsillitis/pharyngitis: clindamycin for 5 days

Toxic Shock Syndrome

▶ Necrotising fasciitis

Toxoplasmosis

Pathogen:
Toxoplasma gondii

Therapy:
- Adults and children (acquisition via transfusion, active chorioretinitis): pyrimethamine (100 mg q12h on day 1, then 25–50 mg/day p.o.) + sulfadiazine 1–1.5 g p.o. q6h + folic acid 10–15 mg p.o. three times weekly; continue therapy until 1–2 weeks after disappearance of symptoms; give folic acid for a further week
- Pregnancy up to 18th week of gestation: 1 g p.o. q8h spiramycin (Rovamycine®, Rovamicina®)

- Cerebral toxoplasmosis in AIDS: pyrimethamine (200 mg p.o. q24h, then 75–100 mg p.o.) + sulfadiazine 1–1.5 g p.o. q6h + folic acid 15 mg p.o. three times weekly ; continue treatment until 4–6 weeks after disappearance of symptoms; or TMP 10 mg/kg SMX 50 mg/kg p.o. or i.v. in 2 doses for 30 days; then suppression therapy

Alternatives to sulfadiazine: 600 mg q6h clindamycin; atovaquone 750 mg q6h; clarithromycin 1g p.o. q12h; azithromycin 1,5 g p.o. q24h; dapsone 50 mg p.o. q24h

- Suppression therapy: sulfadiazine + pyrimethamine as for acute therapy, but half dosage until CD4 cells >200/µl for 6 months
- Primary prophylaxis (CD4 cells <100/µl + IgG toxo-antibody): cotrimoxazole 160/800 mg/day p.o. or dapsone 50 mg/day + pyrimethamine 50 mg + folic acid 30 mg/week
- CNS or ocular involvement: additional prednisolone 1 mg/kg/day in 2 doses until CSF protein starts to fall or chorioretinitis begins to abate

Tuberculosis

Pathogens:
M. tuberculosis and atypical mycobacteria

Primary Therapy of Organic Tuberculosis:
- Six-month regime (standard therapy): initial phase (2–3 months): INH + rifampin + pyrazinamide (PZA) + ethambutol daily, followed by 4-month stabilisation phase: INH + rifampin daily or INH + rifampin 2–3 times weekly. The 6-month regime is the optimal standard therapy. In case of cavernous processes therapy should last at least 7–8 months. Treat recurrences for 9–12 months. Combination of INH + rifampin + PZA is obligatory. The four-drug combination is indicated in cavernous processes, when more than one bronchopulmonary segment is involved, in haematogenous disseminated tuberculosis, and when INH resistance is suspected

- In intolerance of or known resistance to a component of standard therapy: consider longer duration of treatment (American Thoracic Society/Centers for Disease Control and Prevention/Infectious Diseases Society of America. Am J Respir Crit Care Med. 2005)
- In pregnancy: INH + rifampin + ethambutol for 9 months. Pyrazinamide contraindicated
- Tuberculous meningitis: total duration of treatment 12 months

Atypical Mycobacteria (AIDS):
M. avium-intracellulare complex: (clarithromycin or azithromycin) + ethambutol + (rifabutin or rifampin); (clarithromycin or azithromycin) + ethambutol + (rifabutin or rifampin) + (ciprofloxacin or ofloxacin or amikacin or streptomycin)
Primary prophylaxis in HIV-infected patients (CD4 count <100 mm^3): azithromycin 1200 mg p.o. weekly or clarithromycin 500 mg p.o. q12h or rifabutin 300 mg p.o. q24h; discontinuation after CD4 count >100 mm^3
Secondary (posttreatment) prophylaxis after treatment (necessary in HIV patients): (clarithromycin or azithromycin) + ethambutol.
M. celatum: clarithromycin + ethambutol + ciprofloxacin ± rifabutin
M. chelonae: clarithromycin
M. fortuitum: amikacin + cefoxitin + probenecid for 2–6 weeks, then cotrimoxazole or doxycycline for 6–12 months
M. kansasii: INH + rifampin + ethambutol for 18 months
M. ulcerans: rifampin + amikacin; ethambutol + cotrimoxazole for 4–6 weeks

Remarks:
All antitubercular drugs (except rifampin) should be taken together or at short intervals in the full daily dose, if at all possible following a meal. Rifabutin (Mycobutin®, Alfacid®) can be given instead of rifampin. In tuberculosis 300 mg/day p.o. (children: 5 mg/kg/day); in *Mycobacterium avium* infection higher dosage of rifabutin might be needed (450–600 mg/day).

For treatment of *Mycobacterium tuberculosis* exposure and treatment of latent infection with *M. tuberculosis* (formerly known as "prophylaxis") with INH, consult expert (MMWR Dec 16 2005)

Ulcer (Peptic)

Pathogen:
Helicobacter pylori

Primary Therapy:
Preprandial omeprazole 20 mg q12h + postprandial amoxicillin 1 g q12h + clarithromycin 500 mg q12h (p.o.) for 7–14 days

Alternatives:
Preprandial omeprazole 20 mg q12h + postprandial clarithromycin 500 mg q12h + metronidazole 400–500 mg q12h (p.o.) for 7 days

If Treatment Fails:
If possible, await antibiogram (resistance rates over 50%). Otherwise, try omeprazole 20 mg q12h + bismuthate 120 mg q6h + tetracycline 500 mg q6h + metronidazole 400 mg q8h for 7 days

Remarks:
If indicated, noninvasive eradication check 6 weeks after end of therapy

Urethritis (Nonspecific), Nongonorrheal

Most Frequent Pathogens:
Chlamydiae, mycoplasmas, trichomonads, enterobacteria

Primary Therapy:
Doxycycline for 1 week or one single dose of 1 g azithromycin p.o.

Alternatives:
Erythromycin (500 mg/day q6h for 7 days), metronidazole for trichomonads (2 g p.o. as single dose); quinolones in suspicion of enterobacteria (Gram staining!)

Remarks:
In case of chlamydiae, mycoplasmas and trichomonads treat partner!

Urinary Tract Infections

Most Frequent Pathogens:
E. coli, other enterobacteria, enterococci, *Staphylococcus saprophyticus* (young women and children)

Primary Therapy:
- Adults and children: cotrimoxazole, trimethoprim or other sulfonamide/TMP combinations (only when local resistance rate in E. coli <20%; without pretreatment with cotrimoxazole), fosfomycin (3 g as single dose in women) or oral cephalosporins; in most cases of uncomplicated UTI 3 days of treatment suffices, in pregnant women 7 days, in pyelonephritis (▶ Pyelonephritis) 14 days.

Alternatives:
- Adults: quinolones (groups I and II; monitor local resistance)

Remarks:

- Microscopic and bacteriologic examination of urine 3–5 days after starting chemotherapy (urine should be sterile)
- Catheter-related urinary tract infection: systemic antimicrobial prophylaxis should not be routinely used in patients with urinary catheter. Seven days is the recommended duration of antimicrobial treatment in patients with catheter-related UTI who have prompt resolution of symptoms and 10–14 days for those with a delayed response. A 5-day regimen of levofloxacin may be considered only in patients who are not severely ill. A 3-day antimicrobial regimen may be considered for women aged <65 years without upper urinary tract symptoms after a catheter has been removed
- Chronic recurring UTI: microscopic and bacteriologic examination of urine weekly until 3 weeks after end of treatment, then monthly for 3 months, then 3 times at intervals of 6 months
- Chronic recurring UTI (recurrence only 3 weeks after discontinuation of chemotherapy, in frequent reinfection, vesicoureteral reflux without ostial anomaly, obstructive lesions of urinary tract possible), reinfection (≥2 in 6 months) prophylaxis: cotrimoxazole (80 mg TMP/400 mg SMX p.o.) once daily (preferably after dinner) or three times weekly or trimethoprim 100 mg p.o. once daily or cefalexin/ciprofloxacin 250 mg p.o. once daily or nitrofurantoin 50–100 mg p.o. once daily or fosfomycin 3 g p.o. every 10 days, all regimens for 6 months
- Infants: exclude obstructive UTI; in UTI without sepsis only half the usual parenteral dose of antibiotic necessary. Always exclude urosepsis! Blood cultures!

Vaginitis

Most Frequent Pathogens:
a) Bacterial vaginitis: *Gardnerella vaginalis*, anaerobes, mycoplasmas
b) Vulvovaginal candidiasis: *Candida albicans*, other *Candida* species
c) Trichomoniasis: *Trichomonas vaginalis*

Primary Therapy:
a) Metronidazole 400–500 mg p.o. q12h for 7 days or vaginal cream
b) Fluconazole 150 mg p.o. as single dose
c) Metronidazole 2 g p.o. as single dose

Alternatives:
a) Clindamycin 300 mg p.o. q12h for 7 days or vaginal cream
b) Itraconazole 200 mg p.o. q12h (1 day)
c) Metronidazole 400–500 mg q12h for 7 days; tinidazole 500 mg q6h (1 day)

Remarks:
- Trichomoniasis and bacterial vaginitis: foul-smelling discharge, pH >4.5
- Candidiasis: odourless, cheesy discharge, pH <4.5
- In trichomoniasis, always treat the partner (metronidazole 2 g as single dose)
- In bacterial vaginitis and candidiasis: treat partners only if they show symptoms
- Reinfection or recurrence prophylaxis for candidiasis (≥4 episodes/year): fluconazole 100 mg/week or clotrimazole as vaginal suppository 500 mg/week, each for 6 months
- Alternative local treatments: azole derivatives in candidiasis (nystatin less effective); paromomycin in trichomoniasis; clindamycin in bacterial vaginitis

11 Treatment of the Most Frequent Types of Bacterial Endocarditis

Unknown pathogen (native valves)		
Ampicillin	3–4 g	q6h (until pathogen identified)
plus		
Flucloxacillin	4 g	q8h (or oxacillin q6h)
plus		
Gentamicin	1–1.5 mg/kg	q8h
In penicillin allergy		
Vancomycin	15 mg/kg	q12h (until pathogen identified)
plus		
Gentamicin	1–1.5 mg/kg	q8h
Unknown pathogen (artificial valves)		
Vancomycin	15 mg/kg	q12h (until pathogen identified)
plus		
Gentamicin	1–1.5 mg/kg	q8h
plus		
Rifampicin	300 mg p.o.	q12h
Viridans streptococci (native and artificial valves)		
MIC <0.125 µg/ml		
Penicillin G	5 million IU	q6h for 4 weeks
or		
Ceftriaxone	2 g	q24h for 4 weeks

or

| Penicillin G plus | 5 million IU | q6h for 2 weeks |
| Gentamicin | 1 mg/kg | q8h for 2 weeks |

Viridans streptococci (native and artificial valves)
MIC ≥0.125 ≤0.5 µg/ml

| Penicillin G plus | 5 million IU | q6h for 4 weeks |
| Gentamicin | 1–1.5 mg/kg | q8h for 2 weeks |

Viridans streptococci (native and artificial valves)
MIC >0.5 µg/ml

| Ampicillin plus | 3–4 g | q6h for 4–6 weeks |
| Gentamicin | 1–1.5 mg/kg | q8h for 4–6 weeks |

In penicillin allergy and MIC ≤ 0.5 µg/ml

| Vancomycin | 15 mg/kg | q12h for 4 weeks |

In penicillin allergy and MIC >0.5 µg/ml

| Vancomycin plus | 15 mg/kg | q12h for 4–6 weeks |
| Gentamicin | 1–1.5 mg/kg | q8h for 4–6 weeks |

Enterococci (native and artificial valves)
Ampicillin-sensitive, gentamicin MIC >500 µg/ml (high level)

| Ampicillin | 3–4 g | q6h for 8–12 weeks |

Ampicillin-sensitive, gentamicin MIC <500 µg/ml (low level)

Ampicillin	3–4 g	q6h for 4–6 weeks
plus		
Gentamicin	1–1.5 mg/kg	q8h for 4–6 weeks

Ampicillin-resistant, gentamicin-sensitive or penicillin allergy

Vancomycin	15 mg/kg	q12h for 4–6 weeks
plus		
Gentamicin	1–1.5 mg/kg	q8h for 4–6 weeks

Staphylococci (native valves)

Methicillin-sensitive (S. aureus, S. epidermidis)

Flucloxacillin	1.5–2 g	q4h (or Oxacillin 2g q6h) for 4–6 weeks[1]
plus		
Gentamicin	1–1.5 mg/kg	q8h for 3–5 days[2]
or		
Cefazolin	2 g	q8h for 4–6 weeks[1]
plus		
Gentamicin	1–1.5 mg/kg	q8h for 3–5 days[2]

Methicillin-resistant (S. aureus, S. epidermidis) or penicillin allergy

Vancomycin	15 mg/kg	q12h for 4–6 weeks

In vancomycin allergy

Daptomycin	6–9 mg/kg	g24h for 6 weeks

Staphylococci (artificial valves)

Methicillin-sensitive (S. aureus, S. epidermidis)

Flucloxacillin	1.5–2 g	q4h for 6 weeks
plus		
Rifampicin	300 mg p.o.	q8h for 6 weeks
plus		
Gentamicin	1–1.5 mg/kg	q8h for 2 weeks

Methicillin-resistant (S. aureus, S. epidermidis) or penicillin allergy

Vancomycin	15 mg/kg	q12h for 6 weeks
plus		
Rifampicin	300 mg p.o.	q8h for 6 weeks
plus		
Gentamicin	1–1.5 mg/kg	q8h for 2 weeks

HACEK[3]

Ceftriaxone	2 g	q24h for 4 weeks
or		
Ampicillin	3 g	q6h for 4 weeks
plus		
Gentamicin	1–1.5 mg/kg	q8h for 4 weeks

[1] If tricuspid valve affected, 2 weeks' therapy sufficient

[2] Aminoglycoside administration optional

[3] Haemophilus, Actinobacillus, Cardiobacterium, Eikenella, Kingella

Remarks
- Negative blood cultures: consider HACEK, coxiellae, bartonellae, psittacosis, brucellosis
- Fungal endocarditis: amphotericin B ± azole derivative; early surgical intervention necessary

12 Minimal Duration of Treatment for Bacterial Infections

Disease	Duration of Therapy (Days)
Arthritis	14–21
Borreliosis	14–28
Bronchitis	5–10
Brucellosis	42
Cholecystitis	7
Diphtheria	7–14
Diverticulitis	7–10
Endocarditis[1]	14–42
Erysipelas	10
Gonorrhoea	1–7
Meningitis[1]	7–14
– Listeriosis	21
Osteomyelitis, acute	28–42
Osteomyelitis, chronic	180
Otitis media	5–10
Pericarditis	28
Peritonitis	5–14
Pertussis	14
Pneumonia, community-acquired	5–10
– Staphylococci	28
– Pneumocystis	21
– Pseudomonas	21

Disease	Duration of Therapy (Days)
– Legionellae	7–14
Prostatitis, acute	10–14
Prostatitis, chronic	42
Pyelonephritis	14
Salpingitis	10–14
Sepsis	10–14
– S. aureus	28
Sinusitis	5–10
Tonsillitis/scarlet fever	5–10
Ulcer	7
Urethritis	7
Urinary tract infection	3

[1] According to etiology (▶ Endocarditis)

Note:
This table merely provides guidance to the minimum or average duration of treatment for the diseases listed. Rule of thumb for minimum therapy duration: until 3 days after normalisation of temperature and clinical improvement. If 3–4 days of treatment bring no clinical improvement or lowering of fever, then discontinue/change the treatment or doubt the diagnosis.

The longer an antibiotic is given, the greater the risk of pathogen selection, development of resistance or superinfection (e.g. with fungi!). If a treatment is identified as unnecessary, it should be discontinued immediately (!) and need not – e.g. to avoid development of resistance – be given for a total of ca. 5 days.

13 Failure of Antibiotic Therapy

The reasons for failure to achieve the goal of antibiotic treatment can be summarised under three headings:

The Patient
- Weakened autoimmune defence system (cytostatic therapy, cancer, diabetes, alcoholism, liver cirrhosis etc.); foreign bodies (intravenous catheter, bladder catheter, hydrocephalus valve, tracheal tube)
- Abscess or poorly accessible infection site
- Drug fever (fever does not subside!)
- The patient does not take the antibiotic (up to 30%!)

The Pathogen
- The microbe isolated is not the cause of infection (incorrect sampling, incorrect transport, polymicrobial infection)
- Viral infection, fungal infection!
- Mixed infection, or the isolated bacterium is only a contaminant
- Superinfection (hospital infection, fungi!)
- Development of resistance (relatively infrequent)
- Selection of resistant portions of the pathogen population
- Change of pathogen during therapy (especially fungal infection)

The Antibiotic
- Incorrect dosage or administration
- Poor penetration to infection site
- Inactivation of the antibiotic by infusion fluid or simultaneously administered medications
- Antagonism of antibiotic combinations
- Insufficient duration of therapy (e.g. changing antibiotic every 2 days)
- Incorrect resistance data from the laboratory (as many as 20% of cases!)

14 Fever of Unknown Origin: Differential Diagnosis

Definition:
- Fever lasting more than 3 weeks
- Temperature >38.3 °C (several measurements)
- Cause still undetermined after 3 days in hospital

Around 30% of patients with "fever of unknown origin (FUO)" die of the undetected disease. Therefore, the diagnosis "FUO" has to be taken seriously!

Most Frequent Causes
- Infections 25%
- Neoplasms 15%
- Immune diseases 25%
- Unclear 30%
- Miscellaneous diseases 5%

The patients can usefully be divided into **three age groups**:
- <6 years: principally infections of the upper respiratory tract, urinary tract infections and systemic viral infections
- 6–14 years: mainly gastrointestinal tract infections and collagenoses
- >14 years: primarily infections, neoplasms, and rheumatological or autoimmune diseases

I Infections

Common bacterial infections

Abscesses	Liver, spleen, pancreas, subphrenic, true pelvis, prostate, appendicitis, Crohn's disease, diverticulitis
Endocarditis	Rheumatic fever, surgical or diagnostic procedures Important: take several blood samples for culture, because even small doses of antibiotics can inhibit growth of the pathogen! In "culture-negative" endocarditis, look for HACEK, chlamydiae, Coxiella burnetii and Bartonella!
Biliary tract infections	Cholangitis, cholecystitis, bile empyema or infection of the pancreatic duct
Buccal cavity/upper respiratory tract	Dental abscesses, sinusitis
Osteomyelitis	Osteomyelitis of the spinal column, mandible, and maxilla and infections of joint prostheses can display only slight symptoms or none at all
Tuberculosis	The most frequently isolated pathogen in fever of unknown origin (particularly in immune-deficient patients). Some patients only have a fever, without radiographic signs of TB. Negative tine test in generalised infection

Viral infections

	The most frequent pathogens are Epstein–Barr virus (EBV), cytomegalovirus (CMV), hepatitis B virus (HBV), HIV, herpes simplex and parvovirus B19

Less common infections

Amebiasis	Encountered worldwide (hotter countries)
Borreliosis	Tick bites
Brucellosis	Slaughterhouse workers, veterinarians, zookeepers, cooks, laboratory infections
Chlamydial infections	Handling of certain species of bird
Cat scratch fever	Contact with cats
Leishmaniasis	Asia, tropics, Mediterranean countries
Leptospirosis	Second and third phases of disease: pathogen not detectable in blood ± fever as sole symptom
Listeriosis	Haemodialysis patients, after kidney transplant, in tumours of the leukopoietic system, elderly individuals with longer-term corticosteroid therapy
Malaria	Residence or travel in malarial areas (inadequate prophylaxis)
Fungal infections	Residence or travel in endemic areas: coccidioidomycosis (North and South America), histoplasmosis (North America); in immune-deficient patients: systemic Candida albicans infection, aspergillosis, cryptococcosis

Less common infections (continued)	
Rickettsiosis	Tick or mite bites, in Q-fever transmission from pets or airborne (e.g. from infected wool)
Toxoplasmosis	Contact with cats, consumption of raw meat, immunodeficiency
Trypanosomiasis	Residence or travel in central and eastern Africa
Tularaemia	Hunters, foresters, farm workers, dealers in game animals, fur and pelt processors, kitchen staff

II Neoplasms
Hodgkin's disease, non-Hodgkin lymphoma, myelodysplastic syndrome, leukaemia, solid tumour (especially bronchial, pancreas, colon, hepatic cell and renal cell carcinomas)

III Collagenovascular Diseases
Rheumatic fever, lupus erythematosus and other collagenoses, rheumatoid arthritis, Still's disease, temporal arteriitis, periarteritis nodosa, Wegener's disease and other vasculitides, and Crohn's disease

IV Other Causes
Drug fever (!), multiple pulmonary emboli, thrombophlebitis, haematoma, hepatitis, adrenal insufficiency, thyroiditis, sarcoidosis, unspecific pericarditis, thermoregulatory disturbances

V Psychogenic Fever
Habitual hyperthermia, artificial fever

Diagnosis
- Observation of fever course
- Anamnesis (family history, residence or travel abroad, intake of certain medications, alcohol abuse, surgery, exposure to TB, contact with animals)

- Physical examination
- Laboratory parameters
- Noninvasive diagnostic measures (e.g. chest radiography)
- Exclude drug fever. Definition: Fever that arises on administration of a drug and vanishes after its discontinuation, almost always within 48–72 h, in the absence of another cause. The interval between first intake of the drug and the onset of fever varies widely among different groups of drugs: ca. 8 days for antibiotics, ca. 45 days for cardiac medications

Most frequent causes of drug fever:
(alphabetically listed)
- Amphotericin B
- Ampicillin
- Antiallergics
- Antithrombin III
- Atropin sulfate
- Bleomycin sulfate
- Calcium dobesilate
- Carbimazole
- Carbamazepine
- Cephalosporins
- Chinidin
- Chlorpromazine
- Colistin
- Diltiazem
- Diphenyldantoin
- Dobutamine
- Famotidine
- Filgastrim
- Fludarabin
- Halothan
- Hyoscyamin
- Levothyroxin
- Methyldopa
- Minocycline
- Nifedipine
- Nitrofurantoin

- Oxprenolol
- Pamidronat
- Pegaspargase
- Penicillin G
- Pentazocin
- Procainamide
- Procarbazine
- Propicillin
- Ranitidin
- Streptomycin
- Sulfamethizol
- Teicoplanin
- Ticarcillin/Clavulanate
- Tricyclic antidepressives
- Vancomycin

Important Physical Examinations

Lymph nodes:
Repeated palpation of all nodes is crucial, because many diseases cause swelling of the lymph nodes, and sometimes only one single node is involved (Hodgkin's disease, toxoplasmosis, infectious mononucleosis). Particularly the cervical lymph nodes tend to be enlarged in lymphomas or infectious mononucleosis

Ocular investigation:
Exhaustive ocular examination is essential even in patients with no ocular symptoms. The most important findings are the following:
- **Ptosis** in retro-orbital granulomatosis (e.g. Wegener's granulomatosis)
- **Scleritis, uveitis** in rheumatoid arthritis, lupus erythematosus and other collagenoses
- **Conjunctival lesions** in systemic infections (especially in viral and chlamydial infections)
- **Conjunctival petechiae** in endocarditis and lymphomas
- **Conjunctivitis** in tuberculosis, syphilis, tularaemia, mycotic infections (especially in histoplasmosis)

- **Retinitis** in toxoplasmosis and CMV infections
- **Roth's spots on the retina** infectious endocarditis and leukaemias
- **Choroid lesions** in tuberculosis and fungal infections

Examination of skin and mucosae:
Osler's nodes and petechiae of the gums in endocarditis, roseolae of the abdominal skin in salmonellosis, hyperpigmentation in Whipple's disease, skin metastases of various solid tumours and in lymphomas, cutaneous vasculitis in rheumatologic diseases

Laboratory parameters:
The most important laboratory investigations are differential blood count, urine culture, electrolytes, liver function tests, pancreas function tests and blood cultures. More than three blood cultures within 24 h are meaningful only in the case of endocarditis in patients with a prosthetic heart valve and preceding antibiotic therapy. Further materials that may be sampled for investigation are sputum, tracheal secretions and stool. Depending on circumstances these may need to be obtained repeatedly. Nonspecific parameters include BSG, fibrinogen, haptoglobin, CRP, ceruloplasmin and neutrophil granulocytes (all raised). Iron and zinc are lower than normal. Eosinophilia or exanthema occur only in about 20% of cases. Check immunological diagnostic parameters. Elevated lactate dehydrogenases (LDH) and copper (Cu^{2+}) point to haematological neoplasms

Other indispensable investigations:
- Inspection of the head (temporal or cranial arteriitis)
- Inspection of the ocular fundus
- Inspection of the conjunctiva (petechiae)
- Inspection of the finger- and toenails (endocarditis)
- Inspection of the perineal region (fistulas)
- Meningism
- Palpation of all lymph nodes (carcinoma, Hodgkin's disease, HIV)

- Examination of the joints (arthritis)
- Palpation of the thyroid gland (sensitivity indicates subacute thyroiditis)
- Palpation of the spleen (endocarditis, lymphoma)
- Palpation of the liver (pain indicates an abscess)
- Rectal examination and investigation of the true pelvis
- Pressure on the nasal sinuses (sinusitis)
- Auscultation of the heart (endocarditis, idiopathic pericarditis) and the lungs

Further diagnostic measures:
- Radiography (thoracic radiographs should be obtained at regular intervals), ultrasound, and CT/MRI of the abdomen
- Bone marrow biopsy
- Liver biopsy
- Temporal artery biopsy

Skin testing:
Every patient with fever of unknown origin should have a Mendel–Mantoux test and Quantiferon TB test

15 Dosage of Antibiotics in Impaired Renal Function

Joachim Böhler, German Clinic for Diagnostics, Wiesbaden, Germany

Principles:

Individual variation: Even when following the dosage tables, some patients can always show divergent serum concentrations, since metabolism, excretion, albumin binding, etc. can vary markedly on an individual basis. Particularly substances with a narrow therapeutic range (e.g. aminoglycosides) must be closely monitored.

Children: The dosage tables are constructed for adults with steady-state impairment of renal function. Therefore, they are generally not valid for children.

Elderly patients: In old age the glomerular filtration rate decreases, and with it the excretion of many antibiotics. The dosages given for adults are valid up to the age of around 65 years. All dosages can be reduced by 10% in patients over 65, by 20% in those over 75, and by 30% in those over 85. More exact dosages can be derived by calculating the glomerular filtration rate (creatinine clearance).

Estimation of creatinine clearance (CrCl): A 24-h urine sample for calculation of creatinine clearance is rarely available and is usually not necessary for dose adaptation of antibiotics. In patients over 60 years of age or with creatinine >1 mg/dl or with body weight (BW) under 60 kg, however, it is indispensable to estimate the CrCl by means of the stable serum creatinine level (mg/dl) according to Cockroft and Gault:

$$\text{Creatinine clearance} = \frac{140 - \text{age}}{\text{serum creatinine}} \times \frac{\text{BW}}{72} \ (\times\ 0.85 \text{ for women})$$

Note:

1. The estimation of creatinine clearance is mandatory for the determination of maintaining dose of antibiotics. Calculation of dosage derived from serum creatinine is inappropriate since height, weight and gender influence the creatinine value. At a serum creatinine level of 1 mg/dl a 20-year-old man has a CrCl of 120 ml/min, but a 90-year-old man has a CrCl of 50 ml/min! A cachectic 90-year-old man weighing only 36 kg has a CrCl of only 25 ml/min! In a woman of the same age and weight the muscle mass is 15% lower, so the CrCl is 25×0.85=21.25 ml/min.

2. Alternatively the MDRD equation is used by many laboratories for creatinine clearance calculation. This equation, however, should only be used in cases where the CrCl value is below 50 ml/min. It should not be used for CrCl values within the normal range because this would lead to CrCl underestimation and therefore underdosage of the antibiotic. Many laboratory reports include "CrCl (MDRD: 4-variable Modification of Diet in Renal Disease)". These CrCl values can also be used at a CrCl <50 ml/min.

Note:

The most frequent overdosages are those where serum creatinine is "almost normal" and the CrCl is falsely estimated as "normal=100 ml/min".

Note:

Only stable serum creatinine values should be used. Even in anuria (CrCl=0 ml/min) serum creatinine rises by only 1–1.5 mg/dl per day. Although the CrCl is obviously zero, the creatinine level (albeit rising) may be as little as 2 mg/dl!

Rules for dose adaptation in renal insufficiency:

- **Renal and/or hepatic elimination:** The maintenance dose must be reduced for antibiotics that are eliminated largely renally rather than mostly via the liver.
- **Initial dose unchanged:** The size of the first dose of a medicinal drug depends on its distribution volume (e.g. 2 mg/kg

BW), not on the (intact or reduced) excretion. Therefore the first dose of nearly all drugs is the same in patients with and without impairment of renal function! Exception: For aminoglycosides, the nowadays usual single daily dose (e.g. a 400-mg bolus of netilmicin once daily in patients with normal renal function) already includes the normal elimination. The goal of attaining low trough concentrations (=low toxicity) once in 24 h is thus attained in those with healthy kidneys. In anuria, however, it takes 3–5 days before a low trough level is achieved. In the meantime, the excessively long period of high concentrations may have caused irreversible hearing impairment or kidney damage! In overweight individuals the initial dose (mg/kg) of aminoglycosides should be determined by the normal weight, not the actual weight.

- **Reduce the maintenance dose or increase the dose interval?** From the second dose onward, the decreased renal elimination leads to antibiotic accumulation and toxicity, unless the maintenance dose is reduced or the interval between maintenance doses lengthened. With some substances either method can be used. Often however the mode of action or toxicity of the agent dictates the technique of dose adaptation. The dosage tables take these characteristics of the antibiotics into account. For example, with aminoglycosides the peak concentration correlates with the antibacterial effect, but the value and duration of the trough level correlate with the toxicity. Administration of high single doses is desirable with regard to efficacy, but unacceptable because of the increased toxicity resulting from high levels over a period of several days. The dosing recommendations aim to achieve a low trough concentration by 24 h, or by 36 h at the latest. Repeated measurement of trough concentrations is indispensable.

Remarks on use of the tables

(antibiotic dosage in adults with impaired renal function) in
► Chap. 9

- Tables for adults specify upper dose limits for a patient weighing 70 kg. These limits may be exceeded only in exceptional, soundly justified cases. The dose for a given patient is be calculated as follows:

$$\text{Dose} = \text{dose for 70 kg} \times \frac{BW}{70}$$

Example:

Calculation of the highest dose of ampicillin for a 20-year-old man weighing 105 kg with a plasma creatinine level of 0.8 mg/dl: (► Ampicillin)

$$\text{Maximum dose} = 4 \text{ g} \times \frac{105}{70} = 6 \text{ g (every 8 h)}$$

This calculation is only justified however when the patient is of normal or near-normal body weight, i.e. not obese or cachectic.

16 Antibiotic Therapy in Haemo-dialysis, Peritoneal Dialysis, and Continuous Haemofiltration

Joachim Böhler, German Clinic for Diagnostics, Wiesbaden, Germany

The dosing recommendations for CrCl <10 ml/min/1.73 m^2 in ► Chap. 9 are for dialysis patients with varying degrees of residual renal function. The data for CrCl 2 ml/min/1.73 m^2 are for patients with residual function of ca. 200–800 ml urine/day. The figures for CrCl 0.5 ml/min/1.73 m^2 are for patients with no residual function (anuria). The tables include regular intermittent dialysis (3 times per week).

- Haemodialysis (HD) removes a medication to a significant degree only if the substance has a low molecular weight (<500 Da), low albumin binding and low distribution volume. Additional administration of antibiotic is usually unnecessary if the next scheduled dose is given soon after the dialysis.

Recommendations:
- Once daily administration (1/24 h): give the dose after HD.
- Twice daily administration (1/12 h), HD in the morning: give the doses after HD and in the evening.
  Twice daily administration (1/12 h), HD in the afternoon: give the doses at 8 a.m. and after HD.
- Administration 3 times daily (1/8 h): the drug should be given independent of the timing of HD, one dose after HD if possible.

Table 16.1 gives dosage recommendations for patients who are being treated with intermittent HD.
The **initial dose in column 2** may depend on the distribution volume of the medicinal drug (body weight), but are almost always independent of renal function or the dialysis procedure. The initial dose is often higher than the later maintenance dose. A patient inadvertently given the maintenance dose from the

outset may be underdosed for days! For almost all drugs, the maintenance dose on the day of intermittent HD should be given **after** dialysis. The **maintenance dose on the HD-free day (column 3)** and the **maintenance dose on the dialysis day (column 4)** often do not widely differ, if the daily dose on the HD day is given **after** dialysis. The maintenance dose given in column 4 is valid only if the timing of drug administration (**column 5**) is observed. Many drugs are effectively eliminated if inadvertently given before or even during HD. In such a case he patient may be underdosed unless an additional dose of antibiotic (not included in the table) is given after dialysis!

Table 16.2 suggests dosing strategies for treatment during continuous renal replacement therapy: continuous ambulant peritoneal dialysis (CAPD) or continuous venovenous haemo-filtration (CVVH). The data should not be understood as any more than guiding values, as CAPD patients, for example, frequently display appreciable residual renal function and may need higher doses of medication. If known, the creatinine clearance of the kidneys and of the CAPD can be added and the dose given in ▶ Chap. 9 for impaired renal function can be suggested.

CVVH patients are treated with widely varying volumes of filtrate/dialysis fluid (e.g. 1 l/h or 6 l/h), or the treatment may be interrupted. Here, too, in the case of marked deviation from the usual pattern of treatment, the filtrate volume per minute can be taken as CrCl in order to look up the dose in ▶ Chap. 9. The table assumes a filtrate or dialysate flow of 1.5–3 l/h. The data are valid also for continuous venovenous haemodialysis (CV-VHD). An adequately high initial dose is particularly important in intensive care patients, to avoid underdosing.

Tab. 16.1 Antibiotic dosing in intermittent haemodialysis

Column 1: Name of antibiotic
Column 2: Maximal initial dose (independent of renal function or dialysis!)
Column 3: Maintenance dose in renal insufficiency requiring dialysis (CrCl <10 ml/min/1.73 m²) on a dialysis-free day (dosages predominantly derived from ▶ Chap. 9 of this book)
Column 4: Maintenance dose in renal insufficiency requiring dialysis (CrCl <10 ml/min/1.73 m²) on a dialysis day
Column 5: Timing of dose: in most cases administration after intermittent haemodialysis is advisable

	CrCl <10 ml/min maximal initial dose	CrCl <10 ml/min maintenance dose on non-HD days	CrCl <10 ml/min max. maintenance dose on HD day	On HD day: timing of dose
Amikacin	5–7.5 mg/kg	2 mg/kg/24–48 h Aim for trough level <2 µg/ml	4 mg/kg	After HD
Amoxicillin	0.5–2 g (depending on indication)	0.5–1 g/24 h	0.5–1 g/24 h	After HD
Amoxicillin/ clavulanate	1.2 g	600 mg/24 h	600 mg/24 h	After HD
Amphotericin B	0.6–1 mg/kg	0.6–1 mg/kg/24 h	0.6–1 mg/kg/24 h	As desired

Ampicillin	0.5–4 g (depending on indication)	0.5–3 g/24 h	After HD
Ampicillin/sulbactam	1.5–3 g	1.5–3 g/24 h	After HD
Azithromycin	500 mg	250 mg/24 h	As desired
Aztreonam	0.5–2 g	0.5–1 g/24 h	After HD
Caspofungin	70 mg	50 mg/24 h	As desired
Cefaclor	0.5–1 g	0.5 g/8 h	After HD
Cefadroxil	1 g	500 mg/24–48 h	After HD
Cefalexin	0.5–1.5 g	0.5 g/12 h	After HD
Cefazolin	1–2 g	1 g/24 h	After HD
Cefepime	2 g	1 g/24 h	After HD
Cefixime	200 mg	200 mg/24 h	After HD
Cefotaxime	2 g	1–2 g/12 h	After HD
Cefotiam	2 g	1–2 g/24 h	After HD
Cefoxitin	2 g	2 g/24 h	After HD
Cefpodoxime-proxetil	0.1–0.2 g	0.1–0.2 g/48 h (only after HD)	0.1–0.2 g

Tab. 16.1 (continued)

	CrCl <10 ml/min maximal initial dose	CrCl <10 ml/min max. maintenance dose on non-HD days	CrCl <10 ml/min max. maintenance dose on HD day	On HD day: timing of dose
Ceftazidime	2 g	1 g/24–48 h	1 g/24 h	After HD
Ceftibuten	0.4 g	0.1 g/24 h	0.4 g/24 h	After HD
Ceftriaxone	2 g	1 g/24 h or 2 g/48 h	2 g/48 h	As desired
Cefuroxime	1.5 g	750 mg–1.5 g/24 h	1.5 g/24 h	After HD
Chloramphenicol	0.25–0.75 g	0.25–0.75 g/6–8 h	HD irrelevant	As desired
Ciprofloxacin	400 mg	200 mg/12 h	HD irrelevant	As desired
Clarithromycin	500 mg	250–500 mg/24 h	HD irrelevant	As desired
Clindamycin	300–600 mg	300–600 mg/8 h	HD irrelevant	As desired
Colistin	0.6–1 mg/kg	0.6 mg/kg/24 h	HD irrelevant	As desired
Cotrimoxazole	160/800 mg	160/800 mg/24 h	160/800 mg/24 h	After HD
Daptomycin	4 or 6 mg/kg (depending on indication)	4 or 6 mg/kg/48 h (depending on indication)	4 or 6 mg/kg/48 h (depending on indication)	After HD
Dicloxacillin	1 g	1 g/8 h	HD irrelevant	As desired

Doripenem	500 mg	250 mg/24 h	500 mg/24 h	After HD
Doxycycline	200 mg initial	100 mg/24 h	HD irrelevant	As desired
Enoxacin	400 mg	400 mg/24 h	HD irrelevant	As desired
Ertapenem	1 g	500 mg/24 h	500 mg/24 h	After HD
Erythromycin	500 mg	500 mg/12 h	HD irrelevant	As desired
Ethambutol	20 mg/kg	7.5 mg/kg/24 h or 25 mg/kg only after HD		After HD
Flucloxacillin	2 g	2 g/24 h	HD irrelevant	As desired
Fluconazole	400 mg	200 mg/24 h	200 mg/24 h	After HD
Flucytosine	50 mg/kg	50 mg/kg/48 h (only after HD)	50 mg/kg measure concentration	After HD
Fosfomycin	2 g	1 g/36–48 h	2 g/24 h	After HD
Gentamicin	1.7 mg/kg	2 mg/kg/48 h Aim for trough level <2 µg/ml	2 mg/kg/48 h	After HD
Imipenem/ cilastatin	0.5 g (0.25 g if weight <50 kg)	500 mg/12 h	500 mg/12 h	After HD
INH/isoniazid	5–8 mg/kg	300 mg/24 h	300 mg/24 h	After HD

Tab. 16.1 (continued)

	CrCl <10 ml/min maximal initial dose	CrCl <10 ml/min maintenance dose on non-HD days	CrCl <10 ml/min max. maintenance dose on HD day	On HD day: timing of dose
Itraconazole	200 mg/8 h for 4 days	200 mg/12 h from day 5	HD irrelevant	As desired
Josamycin	0.5–1 g	500 mg/12 h	HD irrelevant	As desired
Ketoconazole	200–600 mg	200–600 mg/24 h	HD irrelevant	As desired
Levofloxacin	250–500 mg	250 mg/48 h	HD irrelevant	As desired
Linezolid	600 mg	600 mg/12 h	600 mg/12 h	After HD
Loracarbef	200–400 mg	200–400 mg/72 h	200–400 mg	After HD
Meropenem	0.5–1 g	0.5 g/24 h	0.5–1 g/24 h	After HD
Metronidazole	500 mg	500 mg/12 h	500 mg/12 h	After HD
Mezlocillin	5 g	5 g/8 h	5 g/8 h	After HD
Minocycline	200 mg	100 mg/12 h	HD irrelevant	As desired
Moxifloxacin	400 mg	400 mg/24 h	HD irrelevant	As desired
Netilmicin	1.5–2 mg/kg	2 mg/kg/48 h; Aim for trough level <2 µg/ml	2 mg/kg/48 h	After HD

Nitrofurantoin	Not indicated	Not indicated	HD irrelevant	Not indicated
Norfloxacin	400 mg	400 mg/24 h	HD irrelevant	As desired
Ofloxacin	200 mg	100–200 mg/24 h	200 mg/24 h	As desired
Oxacillin	0.5–1 g	2 g/24 h (max. 1 g/6 h)	HD irrelevant	As desired
Penicillin G	5 million IU	5 million IU/8 h	5 million IU/8 h	After HD
Penicillin V	1.5 million IU	1.5 million IU/24 h	1.5 million IU/24 h	After HD
Piperacillin	4 g	3 g/8 h	3 g/8 h	After HD
Piperacillin/ tazobactam	4.5 g	4.5 g/12 h	4.5 g/12 h	After HD
Protionamide	6–10 mg/kg	1000 mg 2–3 × week	Unknown	
Pyrazinamide	25–30 mg/kg	30 mg/kg/72 h (after HD)	30 mg/kg/72 h	After HD
Quinupristin/dalfo-pristin	7.5 mg/kg	7.5 mg/kg/8 h	HD irrelevant	As desired
Rifabutin	450–600 mg	300 mg/24 h	HD irrelevant	As desired

Tab. 16.1 (continued)

	CrCl <10 ml/min maximal initial dose	CrCl <10 ml/min max. maintenance dose on non-HD days	CrCl <10 ml/min max. maintenance dose on HD day	On HD day: timing of dose
Rifampicin	600 mg	10 mg/kg (max. 600 mg)/24 h	HD irrelevant	As desired
Roxithromycin	300 mg	300 mg/24 h	HD irrelevant	As desired
Spectinomycin	2 g single dose i.m.	Not applicable, because single dose	50% of the dose is removed	
Streptomycin	5 mg/kg	Aim for trough level <4 µg/ml	5 mg/kg/72 h	After HD
Sulbactam	0.5–1 g	1 g/48 h	1 g	After HD
Teicoplanin	3–12 mg/kg	3–12 mg/kg/72 h	HD irrelevant	After HD
Telithromycin	800 mg	400 mg/24 h	HD probably irrelevant	As desired
Tetracycline	Contraindicated	Contraindicated		
Tigecycline	100 mg	50 mg/12 h	HD irrelevant	As desired

Tobramycin	1.5–2 mg/kg	1–1.7 mg/kg/48 h Aim for trough level <2 µg/ml	1–1.7 mg/kg/48 h	After HD
Vancomycin	15 mg/kg; keep trough level >10 µg/ml	No elimination through low-flux dialysis membranes; with high-flux membranes: 1,000 mg ca. every 5 days	1–1.5 g every 5 days	After HD
Voriconazole	6 mg/kg for 2 doses 4 mg/kg/12 h		HD irrelevant	As desired

Tab. 16.2 Antibiotic dosage in continuous dialysis

CAPD, continuous ambulant peritoneal dialysis (2 l q6h)

CVVH/CVVHD, continuous venovenous haemofiltration/haemodialysis (1.5–3 l/h)

Column 1: Name of antibiotic

Column 2: Maximal initial dose (independent of renal function or dialysis!)

Column 3: Maintenance dose in renal insufficiency requiring dialysis (CrCl <10 ml/min/1.73 m²) during CAPD (2 l q6h)

Column 4: Maintenance dose in renal insufficiency requiring dialysis (CrCl <10 ml/min/1.73 m²) during CVVH or CVVHD (1.5–3 l/h)

	CrCl <10 ml/min maximal initial dose	CAPD max. maintenance dose on CAPD days	Dosage in continuous dialysis or filtration CVVH/CVVHD (1.5–3 l/h)
Amikacin	5–7.5 mg/kg	1.25–2 mg/kg every 24 h Aim for trough level <2 μg/ml every 24 h	5–7.5 mg/kg/24 h
Amoxicillin	2 g	0.5–1 g/24 h	0.5–1 g/12 h
Amoxicillin/clavulanate	1.2 g	600 mg/24 h	600 mg/12 h
Amphotericin B	0.6–1 mg/kg	0.6–1 mg/kg/24 h	0.6–1 mg/kg/24 h

Ampicillin	0.5–4 g (depending on indication)	0.5–3 g/24 h	0.5–3 g/12 h
Ampicillin/sulbactam	1.5–3 g	1.5–3 g/24 h	1.5–3 g/12 h
Azithromycin	500 mg	250 mg/24 h	250 mg/24 h
Aztreonam	0.5–2 g	0.5–1 g/24 h	0.5–1 g/12–24 h
Caspofungin	70 mg	CAPD irrelevant	CVVH irrelevant
Cefaclor	0.5–1 g	0.5 g/8 h	0.5 g/8 h
Cefadroxil	1 g	500 mg/24 h	1 g/24 h
Cefalexin	0.5–1.5 g	0.5 g/12 h	0.5 g/12 h
Cefazolin	1–2 g	1 g/12 h	1 g/12 h
Cefepime	2 g	1 g/24 h	1–2 g/24 h
Cefixime	200 mg	200 mg/24 h	200 mg/24 h
Cefotaxime	2 g	1–2 g/12 h	1–2 g/12 h
Cefotiam	2 g	1 g/24 h	1 g/12 h
Cefoxitin	2 g	1 g/24 h	1 g/12 h
Cefpodoxime proxetil	0.1–0.2 g	0.1–0.2 g/24 h	0.1–0.2 g/24 h
Ceftazidime	2 g	0.5–1 g/24 h	1 g/24 h

Tab. 16.2 (continued)

	CrCl <10 ml/min maximal initial dose	CAPD max. maintenance dose on CAPD days	Dosage in continuous dialysis or filtration CVVH/CVVHD (1.5–3 l/h)
Ceftibuten	0.4 g	0.1 g/24 h	0.2 g/24 h
Ceftriaxone	2 g	1 g/24 h	1 g/24 h
Cefuroxime	1.5 g	750 mg/12 h	750 mg/12 h
Chloramphenicol	0.25–0.75 g	CAPD irrelevant	CVVH irrelevant
Ciprofloxacin	400 mg i.v.	CAPD irrelevant	200 mg/12 h i.v.
Clarithromycin	500 mg	CAPD irrelevant	CVVH irrelevant
Clindamycin	300–600 mg	CAPD irrelevant	CVVH irrelevant
Colistin	0.6–1 mg/kg	CAPD irrelevant	1.5 mg/kg/24 h
Cotrimoxazole	160/800 mg	160/800 mg/24 h	160/800 mg/12 h
Daptomycin	4 or 6 mg/kg (depending on indication)	4 or 6 mg/kg/48 h (depending on indication)	4 or 6 mg/kg/48 h (depending on indication)
Dicloxacillin	1 g	CAPD irrelevant	CVVH irrelevant
Doripenem	500 mg	250 mg 12/24h	250 mg 12h

Doxycycline	200 mg initially	CAPD irrelevant	CVVH irrelevant
Enoxacin	400 mg	CAPD irrelevant	CVVH irrelevant
Ertapenem	1 g	500 mg/24 h	500 mg/24 h
Erythromycin	500 mg	CAPD irrelevant	CVVH irrelevant
Ethambutol	20 mg/kg	7.5 mg/kg/24h	15 mg/kg/24 h
Flucloxacillin	2 g	CAPD irrelevant	CVVH irrelevant
Fluconazole	400 mg	200 mg/24 h	400 mg/24 h
Flucytosine	50 mg/kg	25 mg/kg/12 h	25 mg/kg/12 h
Fosfomycin	2 g	1 g/36–48 h	2 g/24 h
Gentamicin	1.7 mg/kg	2 mg/kg/48 h Aim for trough level <2 µg/ml	1–2 mg/kg/24 h
Imipenem/cilastatin	0.5 g	500 mg/12 h	500 mg/12 h
INH/isoniazid	5–8 mg/kg	300 mg/24 h	300 mg/24 h
Itraconazole	200 mg/8 h for 4 days	CAPD irrelevant	CVVH irrelevant
Josamycin	0.5–1 g	CAPD irrelevant	CVVH irrelevant

Tab. 16.2 (continued)

	CrCl <10 ml/min maximal initial dose	CAPD max. maintenance dose on CAPD days	Dosage in continuous dialysis or filtration CVVH/CVVHD (1.5–3 l/h)
Ketoconazole	200–600 mg	CAPD irrelevant	CVVH irrelevant
Levofloxacin	250–500 mg	CAPD irrelevant	CVVH irrelevant
Linezolid	600 mg	600 mg/12 h	600 mg/12 h
Loracarbef	200–400 mg	200–400 mg/72 h	200–400 mg/24 h
Meropenem	0.5–1 g	0.5 g/24 h	0.5–1 g/12 h
Metronidazole	500 mg	500 mg/12 h	500 mg/8 h
Mezlocillin	5 g	5 g/8 h	5 g/8 h
Minocycline	200 mg	CAPD irrelevant	CVVH irrelevant
Moxifloxacin	400 mg	CAPD irrelevant	CVVH irrelevant
Netilmicin	1.5–2 mg/kg	2 mg/kg/48 h Aim for trough level <2 µg/ml	2 mg/kg/24 h
Nitrofurantoin	Not indicated	CAPD irrelevant	CVVH irrelevant
Norfloxacin	400 mg	CAPD irrelevant	CVVH irrelevant

Drug	Dose	CAPD	CVVH
Ofloxacin	200 mg	CAPD irrelevant	200–300 mg/24 h
Oxacillin	0.5–1 g	CAPD irrelevant	CVVH irrelevant
Penicillin G	5 million IU	5 million IU/8 h	5 million IU/8 h
Penicillin V	1.5 million IU	1.5 million IU/24 h	1.5 million IU/12 h
Piperacillin	4 g	3 g/8 h	3 g/6–8 h
Piperacillin/tazobactam	4.5 g	4.5 g/12 h	4.5 g/8 h
Protionamide	6–10 mg/kg	Unknown	Unknown
Pyrazinamide	25–30 mg/kg	30 mg/kg/72 h	No data
Quinupristin/dalfopristin	7.5 mg/kg	CAPD irrelevant	CVVH irrelevant
Rifabutin	450–600 mg	CAPD irrelevant	CVVH irrelevant
Rifampicin	600 mg	CAPD irrelevant	CVVH irrelevant
Roxithromycin	300 mg	CAPD irrelevant	CVVH irrelevant
Spectinomycin	2 g single dose i.m.	CAPD irrelevant	CVVH irrelevant
Streptomycin	5 mg/kg	5 mg/kg/48 h Aim for trough level <4 µg/ml	5 mg/kg/24–48 h

	CrCl <10 ml/min maximal initial dose	CAPD max. maintenance dose on CAPD days	Dosage in continuous dialysis or filtration CVVH/CVVHD (1.5–3 l/h)
Sulbactam	0.5–1 g	1 g/24 h	0.5 g/12 h
Teicoplanin	3–12 mg/kg	CAPD irrelevant	CVVH irrelevant
Telithromycin	800 mg	CAPD probably irrelevant	CVVH probably irrelevant
Tetracycline	Contraindicated	CAPD irrelevant	CVVH irrelevant
Tigecycline	100 mg	CAPD irrelevant	CVVH irrelevant
Tobramycin	1.5–2 mg/kg	1–1.7 mg/kg/48 h Aim for trough level <2 µg/ml every 24 h	2 mg/kg/24 h
Vancomycin	15 mg/kg keep trough level >10 µg/ml	CAPD irrelevant	Only high-flux membranes are used, thus: 1,000 mg every 3–4 days
Voriconazole	6 mg/kg for 2 doses CAPD irrelevant		Not yet investigated

17 Antibiotic Therapy During Pregnancy and Lactation

Antibiotics are classified into the categories A, B, C, D according to their safety during pregnancy. β-Lactam antibiotics inhibit bacterial cell wall synthesis. Since no comparable metabolic events take place in humans, penicillins, for example, can safely be used in pregnancy. Nevertheless, older members of the group should be prescribed.
Accurate diagnosis is imperative at all times during pregnancy and lactation.

Class A: Safe during pregnancy
Human studies have shown no risk for use during first trimester or later in pregnancy.
Nystatin vaginal

Class B: Safe during pregnancy and lactation: accurate diagnosis imperative
There is no known association with birth defects or pregnancy complications.

Amphotericin B
Azithromycin
Cephalosporins
Clindamycin
Daptomycin
Doripenem
Ertapenem
Fosfomycin
Erythromycin
Ethambutol
Meropenem
Metronidazole
Nitrofurantoin
Penicillins (+ betalactamase inhibitors)
Rifabutin

Class C: Accurate diagnosis imperative during complete pregnancy and during lactation

There is insufficient information or some concerns arising from animal studies, but no confirmation of problems such as birth defects in humans.

Anidulafungin
Azoles
Caspofungin
Clarithromycin
Chloramphenicol
Colistin
Cotrimoxazole
Dapsone
Imipenem
Isoniazid
Linezolid
Micafungin
Posaconazole
Pyrazinamide
Quinolones
Rifampin
Telavancin
Telithromycin
Vancomycin

Class D: Contraindicated during pregnancy and lactation

Should not be used unless there are no better alternatives.
Aminoglycosides
Tetracycline
Tigecycline
Voriconazole

Note:
For Doripenem, only limited clinical data on exposed pregnancies are available.
Therefore, Doripenem should not be used during pregnancy and lactation unless clearly necessary.

18 Antibiotics in Liver Diseases

The following antibiotics should be avoided or used at reduced dosage in patients with severe liver disease:

- Amoxillin/clavulanate
- Amphotericin B
- Azithromycin
- Aztreonam (reduced dosage)
- Caspofungin (reduced dosage)
- Cefotaxime
- Ceftriaxone (reduced dosage in simultaneous renal insufficiency)
- Chloramphenicol (reduced dosage)
- Clarithromycin
- Clavulanic acid
- Clindamycin
- Cotrimoxazole (reduced dosage)
- Dicloxacillin
- Doxycycline
- Erythromycin (particularly erythromycin estolate; reduced dosage)
- Flucloxacillin
- Fluconazole
- INH (reduced dosage)
- Itraconazole (reduced dosage)
- Ketoconazole
- Lincomycin
- Linezolid (consider risk)
- Metronidazole (antabuse syndrome!)
- Mezlocillin (reduced dosage)
- Moxifloxacin (contraindication)
- Ofloxacin (reduced dosage)
- Oxacillin (reduced dosage)
- Protionamide
- Pyrazinamide
- Quinupristin/dalfopristin (reduced dosage)
- Rifampicin, Rifabutin
- Roxithromycin (reduced dosage)
- Tetracyclines
- Tigecycline (reduced dosage)
- Telithromycin (reduced dosage in simultaneous renal insufficiency)
- Voriconazole (reduced dosage)

Important!
To date there have been very few investigations of antibiotic therapy in patients with restricted liver function. The table above therefore cannot be considered exhaustive.

19 Diffusion of Antibiotics in Cerebrospinal Fluid and in Cerebral Abscesses

Good in inflamed and noninflamed meninges	Good only in inflamed meninges
Chloramphenicol	Amoxicillin
Cotrimoxazole	Ampicillin
Fluconazole	Cefepime
Flucytosine	Cefotaxime
Fosfomycin	Ceftazidime
Isoniazid (INH)	Ceftriaxone
Linezolid	Cefuroxime
Metronidazole	Ciprofloxacin
Protionamide	Clavulanic acid
Pyrazinamide	Dicloxacillin
Voriconazole	Ertapenem
	Ethambutol
	Flucloxacillin
	Imipenem
	Levofloxacin
	Meropenem
	Mezlocillin
	Minocycline
	Moxifloxacin
	Ofloxacin
	Oxacillin
	Penicillin G
	Piperacillin
	Rifampicin

Poor or nonexistent even in inflamed meninges

Amikacin
Amphotericin B
Azithromycin
Aztreonam
Cefaclor
Cefadroxil
Cefalexin
Cefazolin
Cefotiam
Cefoxitin
Clarithromycin
Clindamycin
Colistin
Daptomycin
Doxycycline
Erythromycin
Gentamicin
Itraconazole
Ketoconazole
Netilmicin
Penicillin V
Quinupristin/dalfopristin
Streptomycin
Sulbactam
Teicoplanin
Tetracycline
Tobramycin
Vancomycin

Good in brain abscesses

Amphotericin B
Ampicillin
Cefotaxime
Ceftazidime
Ceftriaxone
Chloramphenicol
Cotrimoxazole
Flucloxacillin
Fosfomycin
Imipenem
Meropenem
Metronidazole
Penicillin G
Teicoplanin
Vancomycin
Voriconazole

20 Local Antibiotics

Contraindications for Local Antibiotics
- Wound infections with possible discharge of pus and secretion (e.g. Nebacetin®)
- Abscesses
- Sore throat, pharyngitis, tonsillitis. Almost all medications prescribed for local treatment of sore throat or pharyngitis contain unnecessary local antibiotics or disinfectants (e.g. Broncho-Tyrosolvetten®, Dorithricin® throat tablets, Dobendan®, Imposit® etc.)
- Rinsing out of bladder catheters (e.g. Uro-Nebacetin®)
- Small local scalds and burns (e.g. Teracortril® spray)

Note!
Penicillins, sulfonamides, tetracyclines, framycetin and neomycin should no longer be used for cutaneous infections, because they frequently cause allergies and because most pathogens causing purulent infections of the skin – Staphylococcus aureus, streptococci, Pseudomonas aeruginosa, and other Gram-negative bacteria – have become resistant to them. Neomycin is one of the most frequent causes of contact allergies. Alternatives are tyrothricin, polymyxin (Gram-negative bacteria) or bacitracin, fusidinic acid (Gram-positive bacteria) and mupirocin (staphylococci, streptococci).

Possible Indications for Local Antibiotics
- Impetigo contagiosa
- Purulent conjunctivitis, trachoma
- Chronic purulent osteomyelitis (e.g. gentamicin globules or chains)
- Superinfected eczema

Note!

In very many cases the local antibiotic can be replaced by antiseptics (e.g. Betaisodona® solution, Betaisodona® ointment, povidone–iodine). In local applications, solutions containing polyvidone–iodine can cause burns. This can be largely avoided by diluting the solution 1:10 or 1:100 without any great loss of effect. As long as the solution stays brown after application, it is effective. If the solution becomes decolourised by wound secretion, pus, or blood, it has lost its effect. There is no known resistance to compounds containing polyvidone–iodine. In contrast, increasing resistance can be observed to all predominantly locally administered antibiotics. This is true also for gentamicin (e.g. Refobacin® cream). Broadly speaking, therefore, the choice of antibiotics for local application should be restricted to substances with no or only very narrow indications in parenteral therapy, e.g. bacitracin, tyrothricin, fusidic acid, polymyxin and mupirocin.

21 Prophylactic Antibiotic Therapy

Perioperative Antibiotic Prophylaxis

- **Requirements:** As atoxic as possible, appropriate antibacterial spectrum, as cheap as possible, no reserve antibiotics, no broad-spectrum antibiotics. Never: piperacillin, mezlocillin (and similar substances), quinolones, third-generation cephalosporins
- **Suitable antibiotics:** Basic cephalosporins, second-generation cephalosporins (e.g. cefotiam, cefazolin, cefuroxime), aminobenzylpenicillins with β-lactamase inhibitors (e.g. amoxicillin/clavulanate, ampicillin/sulbactam), isoxazolylpenicillins (anti-staphylococcal penicillins, e.g. flucloxacillin), metronidazole. In penicillin/cephalosporin allergy: for instance clindamycin; in oxacillin-resistant *S. aureus:* vancomycin
- **Duration of administration:** A single dose ("single shot" on induction of anaesthesia) generally suffices for operations lasting no longer than 3–4 h. Second dose intraoperatively, never longer than 24 h. Continuation of antibiotic prophylaxis as long as catheters or drains are in place is expensive and of no proven scientific value. There is no such thing as an antibiotic that will stop a drain becoming colonised! Risks of extended use of antibiotics: bacterial selection, development of resistance, higher rate of side effects
- **Decolonisation:** Recent data show benefit (reduction of postoperative *S. aureus* infection) for MRSA carriers decolonised before cardiac and orthopaedic surgery by use of intranasal mupirocin and chlorhexidine bath
- **Indications**
  - **Gastric surgery (incl. PEG):** second-generation cephalosporins, aminopenicillin/β-lactamase inhibitor; single dose; only in presence of risk factors: bleeding gastric or duodenal ulcer, stomach cancer, inhibited secretion of gastric acids, obesity
  - **Biliary tract surgery (incl. laparoscopic cholecystectomy):** 2nd generation cephalosporins or aminobenzyl-

penicillin + β-lactamase inhibitor; single dose; only in presence of risk factors: age >60 years, obesity, icterus, choledocholithiasis, acute cholecystitis. In ERCP: only in presence of obstruction, ciprofloxacin p.o. 2 h before operation

- **Colorectal surgery (incl. appendectomy):** second-generation cephalosporins + metronidazole, ampicillin/sulbactam, amoxicillin/clavulanate; single dose. No antibiotic prophylaxis in aseptic abdominal surgery without opening of the GI tract
- **Penetrating abdominal trauma with suspicion of intestinal injury:** second-generation cephalosporins + metronidazole as soon as possible. If no intestinal injury is found: single dose; with intestinal injury: antibiotics for 12–24 h; antibiotic administration for more than 24 h is justified only if the operation is performed over 12 h after traumatic perforation
- **Vaginal and abdominal hysterectomy:** second-generation cephalosporins + metronidazole or amino-benzylpenicillins + β-lactamase inhibitor; single dose
- **Caesarean section:** second-generation cephalosporins or ampicillin/sulbactam; single dose; not until after clamping of the umbilical cord
- **Abortion and curettage:** second-generation cephalosporins; single dose; only in presence of risk factors, e.g. genital infections
- **Nephrectomy:** possibly second-generation cephalosporins
- **Transurethral prostatectomy:** ciprofloxacin; single dose; indication questionable if urine primarily sterile
- **Transrectal prostate biopsy:** ciprofloxacin one dose 12h before and 12 h after procedure
- **Fractures close to hip joint, joint replacement surgery:** second-generation cephalosporins or anti-staphylococcal penicillins; single dose
- **Open fractures:** second-generation cephalosporins or anti-staphylococcal penicillins; duration 12–24 h

- **Orthopaedic surgery without implantation of foreign material:** no antibiotic prophylaxis
- **Orthopaedic surgery with implantation:** second generation cephalosporins
- **Cardiac and vascular surgery (incl. leg amputation):** second-generation cephalosporins or anti-staphylococcal penicillins (leg amputation: + metronidazole) or vancomycin (high rate of MRSA); single dose
- **Pacemaker implantation:** second-generation cephalosporins; single dose
- **Neurosurgical shunt operations:** second-generation cephalosporins or anti-staphylococcal penicillins or vancomycin (high incidence of MRSA); single dose
- **Head and neck surgery:** second-generation cephalosporins + clindamycin; single dose; only in contamination during major interventions, e.g. neck dissection, pharyngeal or laryngeal cancer
- **Lung surgery:** second-generation cephalosporins; single dose; determine indications on individual basis

Most Frequent Mistakes

- **Too generous:** There are few operations for which the indication has been demonstrated in randomised controlled trials
- **Too long:** A single dose usually suffices! Never: "as long as catheters or drains are in place" (completely false indication!)
- **Too broad:** Never broad-spectrum penicillins, third-generation cephalosporins, quinolones, fixed antibiotic combinations
- **Too ambitious:** Perioperative antibiotic prophylaxis lowers the postoperative rate of wound infections caused by the most frequent pathogens; it does not prevent all postoperative infections by all pathogens

Table 21.1. Prophylactic antibiotic therapy

Disease	Prophylaxis
Endocarditis	
I. Post rheumatic fever, rheumatic chorea, rheumatic heart defect (also with artificial heart valves)	Benzathine penicillin G i.m. 1.2 million IU every 3 weeks or penicillin V 600,000 IU/day divided into 2 doses p.o. or erythromycin in penicillin allergy (250 mg/day p.o. q12h)[1]
II. Congenital heart defect[2], artificial heart valves Cardiac transplantation or history of endocarditis	Scheme A or B (in penicillin allergy scheme C)

[1] With carditis: penicillin G for 10 years or until age of 25 years
Without carditis: penicillin G for 5 years or until age of 18 years
[2] Cyanotic congenital defects, vascular prostheses

Remarks

Paediatric doses: 600,000 IU benzathine penicillin i.m. q24h (>25 kg) once monthly; 200,000 IU penicillin V p.o. (<25 kg); >25 kg as for adults. Penicillin allergy: 25 mg erythromycin, cefalexin per kg/day divided into 2 daily doses

Dental procedures with manipulation of the gums or the periapical region or perforation of the oral mucosa

Respiratory tract: bronchoscopy with biopsies, abscess drainage, tonsillectomy, adenectomy (especially in patients with suspected infectious process)[3]

Gastrointestinal tract: in infections of the gastrointestinal or urogenital tract, therapy with an antibiotic effective against enterococci (e.g. ampicillin, piperacillin)[4]

Urogenital tract: before elective cystoscopy or other interventions in the urogenital tract in presence of infection or colonisation with enterococci, therapy with an antibiotic effective against enterococci. Before nonelective surgery, therapy with an antibiotic effective against enterococci (preferably ampicillin or amoxicillin).

[3] No endocarditits prophylaxis during bronchoscopy without biopsy
[4] No endocarditis prophylaxis during gastroscopy or coloscopy

Table 21.1 (continued)

Scheme	Adults
Scheme A	Amoxicillin 2 g p.o. (>70 kg: 3 g), 1 h before operation
Scheme B	Ampicillin 2 g i.m. or i.v., 1/2–1 h before operation
Scheme C	Clindamycin 600 mg p.o.; or cefalexin 2 g, cefadroxil 2 g, azithromycin 500 mg, clarithromycin 500 mg each p.o., 1 h before operation; or clindamycin 600 mg i.v., 1/2 h before operation
	Recommendation of the American Heart Association 2007

Children

Amoxicillin 50 mg/kg p.o. 1 h before operation or <15 kg: amoxicillin 0.75 g p.o.; 15–30 kg: amoxicillin 1.5 g p.o.; >30 kg: amoxicillin 2 g p.o. (as for adults)

Ampicillin 50 mg/kg i.m. or i.v., 1/2 h before operation

Clindamycin 20 mg/kg p.o. or i.v. 1/2 before operation; or cefalexin 50 mg/kg i.v. 1 h before operation

Table 21.1 (continued)

Disease	Pathogen
Diphtheria	*Corynebacterium diphtheriae*
Haemophilus influenzae **exposure**	*H. influenzae* B

Prophylaxis	Remarks
Adults and children >30 kg: 1.2 million IU benzathine penicillin G i.m. Children <30 kg: 600,000 IU benzathine penicillin G i.m. Penicillin allergy: 40–50 mg/kg/day erythromycin 7 days	Antibiotic prophylaxis for all close contacts, regardless of vaccination status! Also: booster if last vaccination more than 5 years before; primary immunisation if protection inadequate or absent
Adults: 600 mg rifampin q24h 4 days Children: 20 mg/kg rifampin q24h 4 days Children <1 month: 10 mg/kg rifampin q24h 4 days	*Household:* When ≥ 1 contact person ≤ 4 years of age with incomplete vaccination protection or when ≥ 1 contact person ≤ 12 months of age or when one or more immune-suppressed children (regardless of vaccination status) ▶ prophylaxis for all contacts. When all contacts 4 years with complete protection ▶ no prophylaxis. *Kindergarten/school:* If 2 cases within last 60 days and children with incomplete vaccination protection ▶ prophylaxis for all contacts. If a new case occurs ▶ no prophylaxis *Index patient:* Prophylaxis if therapy with ampicillin; no prophylaxis if therapy with ceftriaxone or cefotaxime

Table 21.1 (continued)

Disease	Pathogen
Urinary tract infections, chronic recurring	Stool flora
Meningococci exposure	Meningococci
Newborn conjunctivitis	Gonococci, chlamydiae
Newborn sepsis	Group B streptococci

Prophylaxis	Remarks
▶ Urinary tract infection	
Adults: 600 mg rifampin q12h p.o. 2 days; 500 mg ciprofloxacin p.o.; 500 mg azithromycin p.o.; 250 mg ceftriaxone i.m. Children: 10 mg/kg rifampin q12h p.o. 2 days; 500 mg azithromycin p.o.; 125 mg ceftriaxone i.m.	Only for close contacts (family, kindergarten, mouth-to-mouth resuscitation, intubation, aspiration, etc.) until 7 days before onset of disease in index case; prophylaxis until 10 days after contact is appropriate
Credé prophylaxis (1% silver nitrate)	Only in high-risk groups
Penicillin G 5 million IU i.v. initially, then 2.5 million IU every 4 h or ampicillin 2 g i.v. initially, then 1 g every 4 h until delivery (at least 2 doses before delivery) Allergy: clindamycin 900 mg i.v. every 8 h	Only in colonised women (vaginal und rectal screening in 35th–37th GW) or in presence of one or more risk factors: birth 18 h, temperature ≥38 °C intrapartum, history of neonatal streptococcal infection, bacteriuria with group B streptococci during pregnancy, high-risk birth (e.g. multiple pregnancy)

Table 21.1 (continued)

Disease	Pathogen
Peritonitis, spontaneous bacterial (SBP)	Enterobacteria, Gram-positive cocci, anaerobes
Pertussis	*Bordetella pertussis*
Scarlet fever	Group A streptococci

Prophylaxis	Remarks
a) Ciprofloxacin 500 mg p.o.; b) Cotrimoxazole (160/800 mg p.o.) for 5–7 days or ciprofloxacin 750 mg p.o./week	a) Patients with cirrhosis and upper gastrointestinal bleeding; b) Patients with cirrhosis, ascites and previous SBP
Adults and children: 40–50 mg/kg/day erythromycin 14 days (max. 2 g/day)	All close contacts, regardless of age and vaccination status; additionally for children: untreated patients are contagious for ca. 4 weeks treated patients during the first 5 days of antibiotic therapy
Adults and children >30 kg: 1.2 million IU benzathine penicillin G i.m. Children <30 kg: 600,000 IU benzathine penicillin G i.m. Penicillin allergy: erythromycin, oral cephalosporins 10 days	Only in contacts with pos. throat swab and only in an epidemic (school, kindergarten, barracks); throat swabs of asymptomatic contacts only in an epidemic

Table 21.1 (continued)

Disease	Pathogen
Splenectomy	Pneumococci, group A streptococci, *H. influenzae*
Staphylococcal epidemic in neonatal ward or epidemic staphylococcal wound infections	*S. aureus*
Syphilis	*Treponema pallidum*

Prophylaxis	Remarks
Adults and children >5 years: penicillin V 250 mg q12h Children <5 years: penicillin V q12h 125 mg q6h; 500 mg erythromycin in penicillin allergy; alternatively in children <5 years: amoxicillin 20 mg/kg/day (simultaneous *H. influenzae* prophylaxis)	*Children:* Pneumococcal and Hib vaccination: pneumococcal booster vaccination every 6 years; penicillin V for 3 years; longer in the case of immunosuppression *Adults:* Vaccination as for children; penicillin V in immunosuppression or underlying malignant haematologic disease; duration of prophylaxis unknown (ca. 2 years) Immediate amoxicillin/clavulanate p.o. (self-medication) if any sign of a febrile infection
Mupirocin ointment for ca. 5–7 days or until *S. aureus* eliminated from nose and throat (in case of failure: repeat topical mupirocin, rifampin + fusidinic acid p.o.)	Only in *Staphylococcus aureus*-pos. nose/throat swab in contacts (especially surgeons, nursing staff) (search for staphylococcal infection in contacts). Isolation of infected and colonised patients; in the case of a body wash, use povidone–iodine soap or octenidine
Benzathine penicillin G 2.4 million IU i.m. single dose, ceftriaxone 1 g i.v., i.m. q24h azithromycin 1 g p.o. q24h	Within 30 days after exposure; however, protection not assured

Table 21.1 (continued)

Disease	Pathogen
Tetanus	*Clostridium tetani*
Tuberculosis	*Mycobacterium tuberculosis*

Prophylaxis	Remarks
250–500 IU tetanus immunoglobulin i.m. (children and adults)	Prophylaxis in injured persons with absent or inadequate protection
Children: INH 10 mg/kg/day p.o.; Adults: INH 5 mg/kg/day p.o.; prophylaxis initially for 3 months; if tuberculin conversion after 3 months, prolong prophylaxis to 9 months	Persons who have household contact with a patient with frank tuberculosis; persons with tuberculin reaction and a severe accompanying disease (silicosis, diabetes mellitus, immunosuppressive treatment, renal insufficiency requiring dialysis, severe malnutrition) [MMWR December 30, 2005 / 54(RR17);1-141]

22 Physical Incompatibility of Antibiotics and Antimycotics in Infusion Solutions

Table 22.1 Physical incompatibility of antibiotics and antimycotics in infusion solutions

Antibiotic	Other Agents
Amikacin	Amoxicillin/clavulanate, amphotericin B, ampicillin, cephalosporins, macrolides, pantoprazole, tetracyclines, vitamins B and C
Amoxicillin/clavulanate	Aminoglycosides, bicarbonate, ciprofloxacin, dextrose-containing solutions, glucose-containing solutions, corticosteroids
Amphotericin B	Antihistamines, electrolyte-containing solutions, penicillin G, corticosteroids, tetracyclines, vitamins
Ampicillin	Aminoglycosides, metronidazole, tetracyclines
Aztreonam	Sodium bicarbonate, metronidazole
Cefepime	Metronidazole, vancomycin, aminoglycosides, caspofungin
Cefotiam	Aminoglycosides, fluconazole
Cefotaxime	Sodium bicarbonate, aminoglycosides, pH >7
Ceftazidime	Sodium bicarbonate, aminoglycosides
Ceftriaxone	Ringer solution, aminoglycosides, calcium, vancomycin, fluconazole
Cefuroxime	Sodium bicarbonate, aminoglycosides, colistin, clarithromycin, fluconazole

Antibiotic	Other Agents
Chloramphenicol	Vitamins B und C, pH <5, pH >7, fluconazole, vancomycin
Ciprofloxacin	Calcium, clindamycin, heparin
Daptomycin	glucose
Doripenem	Amphotericin B, diazepam, propafol, potassium phosphate
Erythromycin	Vitamins B und C, barbiturates, tetracyclines, NaCl solutions
Flucloxacillin	Amino acid-containing infusion solutions
Gentamicin	Penicillins, cephalosporins
Imipenem	Lactate-containing infusion solutions, aminoglycosides
Mezlocillin	Aminoglycosides, tetracyclines, procaine, noradrenaline
Netilmicin	Vitamin B, chloramphenicol, sympathicomimetics, β-lactam antibiotics
Penicillin G	Vitamin B, ascorbic acid, pentobarbital, bicarbonate, lactate, tetracyclines
Piperacillin ± tazobactam	Sodium bicarbonate, aminoglycosides
Protionamide	Rifampicin
Quinupristin/ dalfopristin	NaCl-containing infusion solutions
Rifampicin	Sodium bicarbonate, tetracyclines, other tuberculostatics
Streptomycin	Rifampicin, isoniazid, calcium gluconate, sodium bicarbonate, barbiturates, heparin-sodium

Antibiotic	Other Agents
Sulbactam	Aminoglycosides, metronidazole, tetracyclines, prednisolone, procaine, noradrenaline
Tetracyclines	Ringer lactate, sodium bicarbonate, heparin, penicillin G, barbiturates, vitamin B, cortisone
Tigecycline	Amphotericin B, methylprednisolone, voriconazole, chlorpromazin
Tobramycin	Heparin
Vancomycin	Various incompatibilities (refer to product information)

23 Useful Websites

http://www.escmid.org/sites/index.aspx
European Society of Clinical Microbiology and Infectious
Diseases

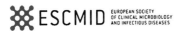

http://www.ecdc.europa.eu
European Centre for Disease Prevention and Control

http://www.rivm.nl/earss/
European Antimicrobial Resistance Surveillance System
(EARSS)

The **EARSNET** is a Europe-wide network of national surveillance
systems providing reference data on antimicrobial resistance
for public health purposes. This network received funding from
the European Commission's Directorate-General for Health and
Consumer Affairs (DG SANCO).

http://ipse.univ-lyon1.fr
http://helics.univ-lyon1.fr
Hospital in Europe Link for Infection Control through Surveillance (HELICS)/
Improving Patient Safety in Europe (IPSE)

  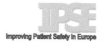

Improving Patient Safety in Europe

HELICS is an international network aiming at the collection, analysis and dissemination of valid data on the risks of nosocomial infections in European hospitals. This network received funding from the European Commission's Directorate-General for Health and Consumer Affairs (DG SANCO). HELICS routine data collection continues to be supported in Work Package 4 of IPSE

IPSE aims to resolve persisting differences in the variability of preventive practices and outcomes with respect to nosocomial infection and antibiotic resistance in Europe. IPSE is a project funded by the European Commission Directorate General for Health and Consumer Protection (DG SANCO).

http://www.eu-burden.info
Burden of Resistance and Disease in European Nations
(BURDEN)

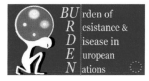

BURDEN is a project that was established to evaluate the dimensions of the economic and societal consequences of antimicrobial resistance (AMR). By exploring the damaging consequences of AMR to individual, hospitals and the health system at large, the project aims to provide realistic estimates of the burden of disease and the costs attributable to infections caused by antimicrobial resistant pathogens for member states and accession countries of the European Union. BURDEN is financed by the EU Commission Directorate-General for Health and Consumer Protection (DG SANCO).

http://www.eu-implement.info
Implementing Strategic Bundles for Infection Prevention and
Managment (IMPLEMENT)

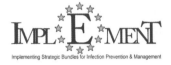

IMPLEMENT is a project designed to provide policymakers,
managers and healthcare workers with the knowledge on the
implementation of improvement measures (bundles) in patient
care for the prevention and management of healthcare-associ-
ated infections in a diverse sample of European hospitals. IM-
PLEMENT is financed by the European Commission's Directorate-General for Health and Consumers (DG SANCO).

http://www.saturn-project.eu/
Impact of specific antibiotic therapies on the prevalence of
human host resistant bacteria (SATURN)

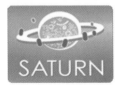

SATURN is a European project started in January 2010 to
study the impact of antibiotic exposure on antimicrobial resistance with a multidisciplinary approach that bridges microbiological, clinical, epidemiological and pharmacological research. SATURN is funded under the 7th FWP (Seventh
Framework Programme).

Subject Index

Printing: Ten Brink, Meppel, The Netherlands
Binding: Stürtz, Würzburg, Germany